Borderline Personality Disorder

A BPD Survival Guide

For Understanding, Coping, and Healing

Anna Nierling

Table of Contents

Introduction

There weren't as many layers between her and the world as there were with the rest of us.

- Renée Knight

I was 10 years old when I realized that my mother was different. One day, she took me and my older brother to the local park to play. We had only been there for what seemed like 20 minutes before she started expressing her disdain for the park.

"Why are there so many people here?"

"We should have come earlier."

"Can you see them staring at us?"

"When will you finish playing? I want to go home now."

That hadn't been the first time I witnessed my mother's mood swings—however, what made me stop and take notice was the fact that other mothers weren't as emotionally vulnerable and restless as mine. Describing borderline personality disorder (BPD), professor and psychologist Marsha Linehan writes, "People with BPD are like people with third degree burns over 90% of their bodies. Lacking emotional skin, they feel agony at

1

the slightest touch or movement" (Goodreads, n.d.).

For someone with BPD, everything always feels too much: Noises are too much. Intimacy is too much. People are too much. They may also feel like their personalities are too much, or that because they are emotionally volatile, they are too difficult to love. My mother would smother us with an all-consuming passionate love one moment, but then the next moment this affection would be too much, so she would withdraw and become emotionally distant.

At first, doctors misdiagnosed my mother's BPD. Unfortunately, this is prevalent in the medical community due to the stigma that surrounds the condition. Many medical professionals seem to debate whether BPD classifies as a mental illness or not, and others go as far as choosing to limit the number of BPD patients they treat.

According to the National Alliance on Mental Illness (NAMI), part of the reason for this stigma has to do with BPD being labeled as a "treatment resistant" condition (Hancock, 2017). However, the treatment outcomes for a patient with BPD have more to do with the doctor's understanding of the symptoms, rather than the condition itself being incurable.

My mother's first diagnosis came back as Bipolar Disorder Type 2. Clearly, doctors had misunderstood her symptoms. She fell into the statistic of the 40% of patients who meet the BPD criteria but are nevertheless misdiagnosed with bipolar disorder (Ruggero et al., 2010). Perhaps this was due to the similarities in symptoms- including mood swings, impulsive behaviors, and suicidal thoughts. However, some common symptoms of BPD such as shame, fear of abandonment, and chronic feelings of emptiness, could not be addressed properly by Bipolar Disorder treatment.

It was only when I turned 20 that my mother received the proper diagnosis. I could sense the relief she felt when a doctor told her that she wasn't crazy and her condition wasn't something to feel embarrassed about. "We are all complicated," the doctor said, "and you can learn to live with your complexities."

It's been decades since my mother began accepting that she had BPD and began learning to live with her complexities. The highs and lows of being raised by a mentally ill mother inspired me to pursue a degree in psychology and dedicate my life to supporting neurodivergent people, helping them to understand and embrace the way their minds work.

The purpose of this guide is to explore BPD: the myths, causes, and treatment options, as well as how BPD impacts decision-making, communication, and emotional regulation. If you are living with undiagnosed or diagnosed BPD, or perhaps you are taking care of a family member who is, you will walk away with up-to-date knowledge, therapeutic techniques, and coping strategies that will help you embrace the condition.

Coping with and building a life around BPD isn't easy—however, learning to do so can help you make peace with who you are and live a meaningful life.

PART 1:

Understanding and Diagnosing BPD

CHAPTER 1:

Understanding Personality Disorders

I'm sorry to be all over the place, my mind doesn't know how to stop, but I'd rather rise up to the insanity, than to further depress on the drop.

\- Vera Hollins

In this chapter you will learn:

- About the three clusters of personality disorders.

- Common risk factors that make you vulnerable to various personality disorders.

Exploring Personality Disorders

A personality disorder is a mental disorder that affects 9% of US adults and 6% of the global population (Cleveland Clinic, 2022). It is characterized by rigid or distorted thinking patterns which affect how you perceive the world and others, as well as your decision-making and emotional regulation skills.

Without having a correct awareness of reality, you are more

likely to feel vulnerable to stimuli in your environment. A loud sound might feel as frightening as hearing a gunshot, being yelled at might cause you to think the other person hates you, and being in an uncertain situation might cause you to act impulsively.

It is also common to think that these behaviors are normal, particularly if you are living with people who are neurodivergent (people who also think differently). You may blame your behavior on other people or situations in your environment, such as thinking that if your family didn't do certain things, you wouldn't resort to thinking or behaving the way you do.

There are various types of personality disorders which are grouped into three clusters based on their similarities. It is possible to display symptoms of one or two personality disorders within the same cluster. You don't need to show all of the symptoms listed under each personality disorder to be diagnosed with it. Let's take a closer look at the three clusters and the personality disorders grouped under them.

Cluster A Personality Disorders

Personality disorders falling under this cluster are characterized by unusual or eccentric behaviors or thinking patterns. The following disorders fall under this category:

Paranoid Personality Disorder

Paranoia is an unshakeable suspicion or mistrust of others, without sufficient evidence to justify being suspicious. People living with paranoid personality disorder often believe that others are conspiring against them.

Symptoms associated with this disorder include:

- Being suspicious of other people's motives.

- Unwarranted belief that others are being deceptive.

- Fear of confiding in others because you believe they will use the information against you.

- Perceiving innocent remarks as insults or threats.

- A tendency to keep score of wrongdoings and hold grudges.

Schizoid Personality Disorder

A personality disorder characterized by a consistent pattern of detachment and signs of disinterest in interpersonal relationships. This pattern may also cause people living with the disorder to show very little range of emotions when engaging with others.

Symptoms of schizoid personality disorder include:

- Little interest in social and personal relationships.

- A tendency to spend time alone.

- An inability to pick up on social cues.

- Being perceived as cold or aloof by others.

- Little interest in sexual activities.

Schizotypal Personality Disorder

Similar to schizoid personality disorder, those who live with this disorder have little to no interest in close relationships and may even feel uncomfortable being around people for too long. Those who do manage to form relationships may struggle to maintain them due to their unusual behaviors and superstitions.

7

Some of the symptoms related to schizotypal personality disorder include:

- Unusual dress sense, thinking, or behavior.

- Illusory perceptual experiences, like hearing voices.

- Social anxiety.

- Believing that they can influence people or situations with their thoughts.

- Behaving as though they are indifferent or being suspicious of others.

Cluster B Personality Disorders

Personality disorders under this cluster are often characterized by overly emotional, dramatic, or unpredictable behavior. People who are diagnosed with any of the following personality disorders will typically express intense and unstable emotions and behaviors.

Antisocial Personality Disorder (ASPD)

People with ASPD tend to show a lack of respect toward others, as well as a reluctance to follow social norms and conventions. They are not afraid to break laws or inflict physical or emotional harm, even if it gets them into trouble.

Some of the symptoms of ASPD include:

- Refusal to take responsibility for unlawful or harmful behavior.

- Showing blatant disregard for the negative consequences of their actions.

- A tendency to deceive others by lying or stealing.
- Repeated criminal violations or trouble with the law.
- Displaying irresponsible and impulsive behaviors.

Borderline Personality Disorder (BPD)

BPD is characterized by low emotional regulation and difficulty maintaining close relationships. People with BPD may also struggle to perceive reality correctly, choosing instead to believe inconsistent thoughts about others.

The following symptoms are associated with BPD:

- Engaging in risky behaviors, like gambling, unsafe sex, or binge drinking.
- Fear of being alone or abandoned.
- Intense and volatile relationships.
- Frequent mood swings, often as a reaction to stressful events.
- Chronic feelings of emptiness.

Histrionic Personality Disorder

People with histrionic personality disorder have a distorted self-image and often experience intense and unstable emotions. In order to feel good about themselves, they depend on the approval of others. When they are not validated, they can react negatively and display dramatic and inappropriate behaviors.

Symptoms of histrionic personality disorder include:

- A strong desire to be validated by others.

- Displaying inappropriate behaviors (like being sexually provocative) to gain attention from others.

- Excessive preoccupation with physical appearance.

- Believing that you have closer bonds with people than you really do.

- Being easily influenced by other people's behaviors.

Narcissistic Personality Disorder (NPD)

NPD is characterized by a consistent pattern of thinking that one is superior to others. People with this disorder tend to have a larger than life personality and they feed off the praise and admiration they receive from others. Underneath this grandiose exterior is often low self-esteem and a lack of true confidence.

The following symptoms are associated with NPD:

- Believing that you are 'chosen' or different from others.

- Fantasizing about gaining power, status, or wealth.

- An inability to empathize with others.

- Being envious of those you believe are better than you.

- Expecting constant affirmation and attention from others.

Cluster C Personality Disorders

Personality disorders that fall under Cluster C tend to produce a sense of fear or anxiety. To escape the perceived threat, people with these personality disorders will turn to the fight-flight-freeze response: They will either act impulsively, develop a dependency, emotionally withdraw, or seek complete control over their environment.

The following personality disorders fall under this category:

Avoidant Personality Disorder

As a defense mechanism against feeling rejected by others, people living with avoidant personality disorder tend to avoid social interactions. This is because they are extremely sensitive to perceived judgment, as a result of their chronic feelings of inadequacy.

Symptoms associated with avoidant personality disorder include:

- Being extremely sensitive to criticism.
- Feeling inferior to others.
- Avoiding group activities that require interaction with others.
- Extreme shyness in interpersonal relationships.
- Fear of embarrassing themselves in front of people.

Dependent Personality Disorder

People with dependent personality disorder have a chronic need to be cared for by others. This might involve taking the submissive role in relationships and behaving as though they are incapable of taking care of themselves. It is common for these people to enter codependent relationships with people who are willing to be their caretakers or enablers.

Symptoms of dependent personality disorder include:

- Being excessively clingy or needy in a relationship.
- Fear of making independent decisions.

- A need for constant reassurance from others.

- Fear of confrontation or making others upset.

- Tolerating poor treatment in relationships due to a fear of being alone.

Obsessive-Compulsive Personality Disorder (OCPD)

OCPD is characterized by the obsessive need for order and cleanliness; this is how people with the disorder regulate their anxiety and feel a sense of control. They may even develop an expectation for perfection, which makes it difficult for them to complete tasks within the allotted time, be present in their relationships, or enjoy the simple pleasures of life.

Some of the symptoms associated with OCPD include:

- Obsessing over small details, processes, or experiences.

- Feeling disappointed when tasks are not completed perfectly, or when people fail to meet your high expectations.

- The desire to control people, situations, and tasks, and feeling anxious when placed in situations or encountering people whom you cannot control.

- Inability to let go of unused or broken items.

- Being inflexible when it comes to your morals, values, and ethics.

Please note that OCPD is a separate condition from Obsessive Compulsive Disorder (OCD), which would be classified as a type of anxiety disorder. People with OCD are aware of their compulsions and the kinds of situations that trigger them. In contrast, those with OCPD are often unaware of their compulsive behaviors and the stressful impact they cause on their lives.

It is common for people to be diagnosed with more than one personality disorder. Generally speaking, it is only during adolescence that personality disorders can be detected: This is because, until then, one's personality hasn't fully developed. Thus, most people only receive a diagnosis after the age of 18, with the exception of antisocial personality disorder, which can be detected as early as 11 years old.

What Causes Personality Disorders?

Since there are so many different types of personality disorders, it can be confusing to distinguish between bad behavior or a negative character trait and a symptom of a personality disorder. To help you identify a personality disorder, keep the following signs in mind:

- **Personality disorders attack your identity and sense of self.** There is a difference between feeling insecure and having a distorted image of yourself. Everybody experiences insecurities from time to time, especially in this modern era of social media. However, when your self-image is unstable, meaning it changes often or may be unrealistic (for example, you think too low or highly of yourself), then this may be a sign of a personality disorder.

- **Due to your inability to self-regulate, your relationships suffer.** It is common to have disagreements with people whom you are close to. However, when the source of conflict is frequently due to your own inappropriate behaviors or the unfounded conclusions you have drawn about people, then the issue isn't about the quality of the relationship, but rather the inner conflict you feel within yourself that is being projected onto another person.

Apart from these two distinct signs, you can also identify a personality disorder based on certain risk factors that make you more vulnerable to this experience. Below are three risks factors associated with personality disorders:

1. **Social and Environmental Factors**

The family or community you grew up in can affect how you develop a sense of identity. Oftentimes, being raised in a dysfunctional home environment or community can expose you to violence, trauma, emotional neglect, and abandonment. Below are some of the social and environmental experiences that can make you vulnerable to developing a personality disorder:

- Living with a mentally ill parent or a parent who has a drug or alcohol abuse problem.

- Having little to no contact with your parents due to their busy work schedules or being taken care of by extended family, such as living with your grandmother.

- Having little to no support after experiencing trauma like rape, bullying, being chronically ill, surviving a car accident, etc.

- Being a victim of poverty and discrimination.

2. **Early Childhood Experiences**

Similar to the first factor, early childhood experiences have a lot to do with how you were raised, the coping mechanisms you adopted, and the type of behaviors that were modeled in front of you. As a way to cope in such a tumultuous environment, you might develop beliefs about yourself and others that shape your experience of reality. Some of the traumatic experiences that can make you vulnerable to developing a personality disorder include:

- Childhood neglect.
- Loss of a parent or someone close to you.
- Witnessing domestic violence.
- Feeling emotionally invalidated by your parents.
- Fear of expressing your thoughts and emotions.

It is worth noting that not all traumatic events will lead to developing a personality disorder. What often makes a trauma survivor vulnerable is the lack of support during difficult times, as well as their conceptualization of their traumatic experiences (the stories they create about what happened to them or how their experiences shaped them).

3. Genetic Factors

Researchers are still investigating how much of a personality disorder is due to the individual's personality and how much of it is a result of genes. Nonetheless, we know that there are aspects of our personality that are hereditary (such as inheriting impulsivity from a parent who is also impulsive, or inheriting an addictive personality).

There is also an argument that some aspects of our personality are due to modeled behavior during early childhood. For example, being raised by a narcissistic parent who uses love as a tool for manipulation can influence how you perceive love or the meaning you ascribe to relationships. Similar to your parent, you may grow up believing that people are objects used for your end

15

goal, instead of respectable individuals who think and feel for themselves.

Chapter Takeaways

Personality disorders are mental disorders that affect how you see yourself and relate to others. These disorders are prevalent in 9% of the US population and 6% of the global population (Cleveland Clinic, 2022). There are three broad clusters of personality disorders, consisting of conditions with similar symptoms and characteristics. It is common to be diagnosed with more than one condition within the same cluster.

Some of the risk factors that can make you vulnerable to developing a personality disorder include the type of environment you grew up in, your early childhood experiences (such as being a survivor of trauma), and inheriting or learning certain behavioral traits from your caregivers.

Now that you have a deeper understanding of personality disorders, we will take an in-depth look at BPD and how it might shape your sense of self, your relationships, and your experience of reality.

CHAPTER 2:

Taking a Closer Look at BPD

[People with BPD] create the vicious circles they fear most.
They become angry and drive the relationship to the breaking
point, then switch to a posture of helplessness and contrition,
beg for reconciliation.

\- Theodore Millon

In this chapter you will learn:

- About the history and latest breakthroughs in our knowledge of BPD.

- What life feels and looks like for someone living with BPD.

The History Behind BPD

BPD was first recognized as a mental disorder in 1980 when it was listed in the Diagnostic and Statistical Manual for Mental Health Disorders, Third Edition (DSM-3) (Optimum Performance Institute, 2014). This doesn't mean that BPD didn't exist prior to that time. However, doctors and researchers had struggled for many years to figure out what caused the condition and its various symptoms.

The earliest record of BPD dates back to 1938, when psychoanalyst Adolph Stern listed many of the symptoms of BPD and called the people who experienced those symptoms the "border line group" (Optimum Performance Institute, 2014). This was because BPD symptoms seemed to be on the border of psychosis and neurosis. From then onward, many doctors attempted to explain the realities of people living with BPD. In the 1940s, Helene Deutsch defined them as people who depended on the personalities of others and Robert Knight linked the concept of ego states with symptoms of BPD.

Anthropologist Roy Grinker is credited for being the first person to lead research into BPD, which was instrumental in helping the medical community understand what the condition was about. In 1968, he published a book called *The Person with BPD Syndrome*, which included a study on patients who were hospitalized with BPD (Grinker et al., 1968). A few years later, psychiatrist John G. Gunderson (known as the "father of BPD") published research about the disorder that helped to get BPD listed in the DSM-3.

Breakthroughs in the Study of BPD

Research into the causes and treatment options for BPD have continued over the years. One of the major breakthroughs occurred about 40 years ago when professor and psychologist Marsha Linehan worked with a group of suicidal women who were diagnosed with BPD.

Many doctors were reluctant to treat these women because they didn't just have one problem, but instead displayed a variety of behavioral issues to treat such as substance abuse, self-harm, and anxiety. Therapists in the 80s didn't really know what to do with these temperamental patients, except to reduce their number of suicidal attempts.

At first Professor Linehan investigated several existing therapies to treat BPD. The first was Cognitive Behavioral Therapy (CBT), one of the leading therapies that was being used to treat BPD patients at the time. She discovered that CBT wasn't effective for people with borderline personalities because of the type of childhoods people with the disorder often experienced.

The focus of CBT is to encourage the patient to recognize and slowly change harmful thoughts and emotions. However, someone with BPD often grows up with a distorted or unstable sense of self, which means that they are not able to distinguish between who they are and the symptoms of their condition. Therefore, treating a person with BPD with this type of therapy is likely to make them feel confused, irritated, and lead to more cognitive dissonance.

Another therapy Professor Linehan looked at was couple's therapy. Since BPD affects how a person relates to others in their relationships, many people with borderline personalities were seeking help from relationship therapists. However, this form of therapy also proved ineffective. The nature of the therapy, which is to get a partner to see the other partner's perspective, would make the individual with BPD feel misunderstood and rejected, and increase their self-loathing.

Observing the suicidal women, Professor Linehan believed they needed a type of therapy that would encourage self-acceptance while holding them accountable to make the necessary improvements in their lives. The two themes that Linehan found necessary were acceptance and change, and, from this understanding, she developed a therapy known as Dialectical Behavior Therapy (DBT). Something that is 'dialectical' has opposing forces, and this was true with the opposing nature of acceptance and change. Nevertheless, these opposing forces are necessary to achieve the four pillars of DBT, which are to build:

- Mindfulness Skills
- Distress Tolerance Skills
- Emotion Regulation Skills
- Interpersonal Effectiveness Skills

DBT was geared toward teaching these suicidal patients fundamental skills to cope with difficult life situations, rather than focusing on changing their thoughts and emotions. They were also not discouraged to think in a particular way, but instead to learn how to accept their negative thoughts and validate their strong emotions. Linehan's colleagues at the University of Washington recorded her sessions so that they could later refine the process of conducting DBT.

Since her clinical trial in the late 90s, there have been over 10 clinical studies that compared DBT with other types of therapy in treating BPD. In comparison, DBT has proven to be more successful in reducing suicide and suicide attempts, in helping borderline patients remain in treatment, and in treating comorbidities like depression and anger management (Promises Behavioral Health, 2011).

Common Symptoms of BPD

BPD can manifest in a number of ways. However, for the purpose of receiving a diagnosis, the patient is required to display at least five out of nine symptoms. These include:

- **Fear of abandonment.** A person with BPD has an immense fear of being alone, whether it is a physical or emotional separation. Even something as normal as a loved one taking longer than usual to respond to a text can be upsetting. The fear of abandonment can lead to desperate behaviors, such as being clingy, begging people to stay, or starting fights just to feel a sense of closeness.

- **Tumultuous relationships.** A common pattern for someone with BPD is to have intense relationships that only last a short while. They may idealize a new friend or lover and display a lot of affection early on, only to push back when the intimacy becomes unbearable. The constant push and pull is what makes relationships move from one extreme to another, and feel unstable or unreliable.

- **Unclear self-image.** Someone with BPD may come across as being confused about who they are. The tendency is to define themselves in extreme terms, such as being either good or bad, without regarding the complexities of their human nature. It is also common for someone with BPD to morph their identity around the people closest to them. This can give the illusion of finally discovering who they are, but this borrowed self-image is not stable or sustainable either.

- **Impulsive behaviors.** A person with BPD will frequently push boundaries, seek novel experiences, and look for the next 'high'. Risky and impulsive behaviors are often what make the person feel a sense of freedom from the emotional turmoil they are harboring inside. In the long-term, these behaviors can be destructive and interfere with daily functioning.

- **Self-harming behaviors.** Another common symptom of BPD is thinking about or deliberately self-harming. This kind of behavior could be motivated by the desire to punish themselves (which stems from self-loathing), or the desire to release the build-up of emotional pain.

- **Splitting.** A person with BPD has a tendency to divide experiences, seeing them as either black or white. People and situations are given positive or negative attributes as a way of explaining why they are that way. Those people or circumstances that are seen as 'bad' are quickly discarded, and those that are seen as 'good' are embraced. Splitting can occur in cycles, which means that someone who was previously seen as good can suddenly switch to being seen as bad, and the process of devaluation and discarding of that relationship ensues.

- **Feelings of emptiness.** It is common to hear someone with BPD talk about feeling empty inside, as though they are living with an inner void. In extreme cases, this feeling of emptiness can cause the person to feel like they are nobody, or that their life means nothing. To avoid this uncomfortable experience, the person may turn to substances or reckless behaviors in an attempt to fill the void.

- **Uncontrollable anger.** Someone living with BPD can experience intense rage and may have difficulty calming down once their anger has erupted. Out of anger, they might become violent and take extreme measures like ending a relationship. Alternatively, their anger can be directed inward, such as when they feel disappointed in themselves.

- **Dissociation.** When feeling emotionally distressed, a person with BPD can mentally disconnect from reality, a term known as dissociation. At first, this may start out as zoning into space (daydreaming), or being absorbed in work or a book. However, other more extreme forms of dissociation may occur, such as becoming paranoid, having amnesia, or experiencing depersonalization (having an out-of-body experience or feeling as though one's environment isn't real).

The symptoms of BPD can also be associated with co-occurring conditions, like anxiety, depression, bipolar disorder, or substance abuse. When these co-occurring conditions are treated, persisting symptoms of BPD can improve. However, it is also true that even when symptoms of BPD are cleared, one can still battle with conditions like anxiety or depression.

Exploring the Mind of Someone Living With BPD

The mind of a person with BPD is often a mystery to doctors, coworkers, friends, and family. At times, the individual may show signs of emotional distress, but even before this experience can be understood, they have somehow recovered and are back to their charming and loveable self. Some will be quick to label this as erratic, impulsive, or irrational behavior, but underneath it all is a deep fear of abandonment.

This fear of abandonment is often associated with early childhood experiences where the person with BPD felt extremely insecure. Their insecurity could have been brought about by the fear of parents leaving, the fear of being rejected, or a feeling of being unlovable. At some point, the person with BPD's insecurity becomes overwhelming, making it difficult for them to separate what is real from what is imagined.

For example, as a result of feeling unlovable, the person with BPD may start to believe that something is inherently wrong with them, as though they were born with some kind of "factory fault" that taints how others see them. Eventually, this may grow to become a deep sense of self-hatred that warps the individual's self-perception (how they see themselves) and makes them more susceptible to self-destructive behaviors.

Therefore, as a result of this chronic fear of abandonment, as well as their deep insecurities and other false ideas about themselves, the person with BPD adopts habits like testing relationships, pushing people away, making impulsive decisions like quitting a good job, or jumping to conclusions about what others are possibly thinking. Similar to narcissists, those with BPD also tend to need excessive amounts of reassurance from others in order to feel safe in relationships. To get along with a person with BPD, friends and family must understand how sensitive this individual is to anything perceived as criticism. Instead of interpreting it as constructive feedback, the person with BPD will see it as a reflection of their personal inadequacy.

People with BPD can create havoc in their relationships, but this has a lot to do with their ideas and beliefs. One of the common signs of the disorder is paranoia, which is the feeling that others don't have their best interests at heart. Since people with BPD already have an unstable self-construct, you can imagine how terrifying that thought would be. The only thing worse than their inability to trust themselves is the inability to trust others. Just like any other human being, people with BPD crave a sense of belonging and to be settled in their relationships. However, the inner voices inside their head create problems where problems don't exist.

What often helps people with BPD cope with their condition is coming to terms with their unresolved emotional wounds—after all, this is where their fear of abandonment began. DBT skills are useful in helping people with BPD slow their minds down, separate themselves from their thoughts and emotions, and recognize the impact of their behaviors on their social and personal relationships. This kind of recognition is the starting point to setting healthy personal boundaries, gaining deeper self-awareness, and learning how to regulate strong emotions.

Chapter Takeaways

BPD was only recognized as a mental disorder in 1980, although the earliest diagnosis was performed by Adolph Stern in 1938, when he identified borderline symptoms in patients and labeled them, "the border line group". Since then, research into the condition has been ongoing, with new discoveries in treatment options like DBT gaining in popularity. Nonetheless, there is still a long way to go before medical professionals understand what is really taking place in the mind of a person with BPD, and provide the kind of support they deserve.

The first step in gaining more knowledge about BPD is debunking common myths associated with the condition. The following chapter will separate the myths from the facts.

CHAPTER 3:

Debunking Myths About BPD

*In practice 'borderline' is almost always used to indicate that
the patient is hostile, demanding, unpleasant, manipulative,
attention-seeking, and prone to regression and dependency if
admitted to hospital; in other words the patient is a witch by
"Malleus Maleficarum" criteria.*

- Colin A. Ross

In this chapter you will learn:

- Why people living with BPD are often stigmatized.

- About the common myths surrounding BPD, as well the
facts needed to debunk them.

The Stigma Surrounding BPD

A stigma can be defined as a preconceived idea that causes
someone to look down upon those who fall under the
stereotype. This often leads to unfair or poor treatment, which is
justified by the stereotype.

People suffering with mental illness are usually stigmatized due to the misinformation surrounding mental health. Instead of learning about various mental health conditions, society or groups of people create preconceptions about mentally ill people, which affect how they behave toward them. For example, poor depictions of mentally ill people in movies have been found to negatively impact how people treat them in real life. Someone might view a mentally ill person as dangerous, irresponsible, helpless, or intellectually challenged.

The stigma surrounding BPD isn't only perpetuated by societal prejudices, but by the medical community also. The lack of understanding about BPD causes many doctors to treat borderline patients with lesser importance or sense of urgency. Some of the common stereotypes about BPD that exist in the medical community are that people with BPD seek attention and create drama for themselves. Therapists who unconsciously hold this negative perception about BPD patients may not take borderline symptoms seriously. Plus, the lack of understanding about BPD can make it harder for therapists to make the correct diagnosis to begin with and prescribe the appropriate treatment.

Perry Hoffman, who is the founder of the National Educational Alliance for Borderline Personality Disorder (NEABPD), noted how BPD was often treated with so much shame and disgust that even those who suffered from it hated their condition. The only other illnesses that fit this category, he remarked, were leprosy or AIDS (Gunderson & Hoffman, 2016).

In order to remove the stigma about BPD, it is crucial that we encourage society at large to gain more understanding about what it is, what causes it, and the most appropriate treatment options. Moreover, we must be willing to debunk common myths that fuel discrimination and instead provide truthful information.

Ten Myths and Facts About BPD

People with BPD tend to feel guilty or ashamed for living with the condition. This has a lot to do with the quality of support they receive from medical doctors, friends, and family. Below are common myths that have perpetuated a stigma around BPD. Below each myth are the facts that are typically bypassed. By unlearning these myths and being empowered by facts, we can all work toward ending the stigma.

1. Myth: BPD isn't a real mental illness.

For over 40 years, the American Psychiatric Association (APA) has recognized BPD as a universal mental health disorder in its publication known as DSM, which it uses to diagnose mental disorders.

2. Myth: BPD only affects women.

Research shows that women are more likely to experience BPD than men—however, it isn't a condition that only affects women. In fact, men statistically make up 25% of people with BPD (The Recovery Village, 2022). One of the harmful consequences of this myth is that men are less likely to come forward and seek treatment for BPD, since they don't believe they can have it or they fear that they will be ridiculed by people if they admit to living with it.

3. Myth: People with BPD seek drama on purpose.

The symptoms of BPD carry harsh consequences for the sufferer, particularly when it comes to their ability to keep a job, regulate their emotions, and maintain healthy relationships. BPD is not a comfortable condition to live with because of the destructive ideas and behaviors it reinforces. No individual would deliberately put themselves under that magnitude of stress, anxiety, and instability.

4. Myth: Suicidal threats made by people with BPD shouldn't be taken seriously.

Making suicidal threats is not a sign of attention-seeking; it is a request for help. It means that to some degree, the individual has contemplated suicide. This should be enough to treat their mental health as a matter of urgency. Research shows that as much as 10% of people with BPD will commit suicide, while a larger number will make several attempts at suicide or engage in self-harming behaviors (The Recovery Village, 2022).

5. Myth: People with BPD aren't capable of showing genuine love.

All human beings are capable of receiving and showing love, and people with BPD are no different. In fact, people with BPD are capable of maintaining long-term relationships, parenting children, and entering fields of work that require interpersonal skills. Their challenges with regulating emotions or managing their behaviors can be addressed with the appropriate treatment plan, which can reduce conflict in their relationships.

6. Myth: Being in a relationship with a person with BPD can be dangerous.

When someone with BPD has not yet received a diagnosis or begun treatment, they can act in ways that are hurtful to themselves and their loved ones. Nevertheless, when it comes to physical or emotional harm, people with BPD are more likely to harm, judge, or punish themselves than they are other people. These attacks may be fueled by feelings of guilt and shame that they have to live with. Getting the right treatment can reduce the intensity of these emotions and bring more stability into the individual's life.

29

7. Myth: BPD is not treatable.

This myth is harmful, not only for the person living with BPD, but also for the doctors who are responsible for treating this condition. There is no doubt that treating BPD requires a number of different interventions—however, there is evidence that certain medications and therapies do work. What's important is getting started with treatment as soon as possible and finding the right options for each individual.

8. Myth: People with BPD are not capable of living independent lives.

It is true that some BPD patients need to be hospitalized in order to receive the care they need. However, not all people with BPD are hospitalized or stay in the mental health system forever. BPD exists on a spectrum, which means that symptoms for each individual can range in severity. Early treatment can prevent the worsening of symptoms and help people with BPD live a stable and fulfilling life.

9. Myth: Living with BPD is a choice.

There isn't anyone living with a mental disorder that chooses to have one due to the amount of disruption it causes to one's livelihood. BPD attacks the mind, but it also interferes with daily functioning, self-image, work, and relationships. The cause of BPD is often related to traumatic childhood experiences, which is also something outside of one's control. Therefore, no one diagnosed with BPD chooses to view life, or relate to others, in that particular way.

10. Myth: People with BPD are not willing to help themselves.

Unfortunately, this myth is perpetuated within the medical

community. Doctors and therapists treating BPD tend to be discouraged when their treatment plans seem to do little work in addressing the condition. What's worse is that the person with BPD's attitude toward treatment can also make doctors believe that the patient isn't willing to help themself. However, there is another way of looking at this, which is that people with BPD have not been taught the kind of interpersonal skills or emotional intelligence skills that make it possible to support their own healing process. Therapies like DBT are able to transfer these skills and increase patient participation in treatment.

Chapter Takeaways

What is common amongst these 10 myths is the level of accountability that doctors, friends, and family expect to see in people with BPD. When little accountability is shown, friends and family might perceive the person with BPD's behavior as rebellious or attention-seeking. However, this is not the case. People with BPD may look and talk like the rest of us, but unlike us, they don't have the psychological tools needed to build and maintain a healthy identity and healthy relationships. If they were equipped with these tools, they wouldn't continue to attack themselves and sabotage their relationships.

Once you have identified the symptoms of BPD, it is important to seek a medical diagnosis. The following chapter will provide you with more information on how BPD is diagnosed.

CHAPTER 4:

The Process of Diagnosing BPD

That was the crux. You. Only you could work on you. Nobody could force you, and if you weren't ready, then you weren't ready, and no amount of open-armed encouragement was going to change that.

- Norah Vincent

In this chapter you will learn:

- The criteria to get diagnosed with BPD.

- Subtypes of BPD, which are not included in the DSM-5.

Scheduling an Assessment

If you suspect that you, or a loved one, may be living with BPD, it is important to schedule an appointment with a medical professional as soon as possible. The doctor will take you through a BPD assessment, which is essentially a screening for BPD symptoms. At the end of the assessment, you will either receive a diagnosis of BPD or be diagnosed with a similar disorder. Since the symptoms of BPD overlap with other mental health disorders, it is possible that what you believe to be BPD is actually something else.

The first step to scheduling an assessment is finding the right medical professional. Look for a doctor who specializes in mental health disorders and who has previously diagnosed and treated individuals with BPD.

Below is a list of doctors that are qualified to offer BPD assessments, diagnoses, and treatments:

- Psychiatrist
- Psychiatric nurse practitioner
- Licensed mental health counselor
- Licensed professional counselor
- Licensed clinical social worker
- Licensed independent social worker
- Clinical psychologist
- Licensed clinical professional counselor

Choosing the right doctor can reduce the likelihood of misdiagnosing BPD or not receiving the quality of care you deserve. Ideally, your doctor should have many years of experience successfully treating BPD patients through various treatment options. Extra brownie points must be awarded to doctors who are trained DBT practitioners and are certified by the DBT-Linehan Board of Certification.

If you are fortunate enough to have health insurance, ask your health insurance provider for recommendations of qualified medical doctors nearby. There may also be public or private mental health programs in your city that offer BPD assessment and diagnostic services.

The assessment process will require you to share personal information about yourself, particularly your medical history, in order for the doctor to make an accurate assessment. The more open and honest you are, the easier it will be for the doctor to assess your symptoms. Some of the questions you may be asked include:

- Current and past symptoms

- Family and work history

- Current life situation

After the assessment has been completed, you will likely receive your BPD diagnosis. There is also the possibility that your doctor may require additional information or testing before giving you a diagnosis. After your assessment, some doctors may refer you to another specialist for a second opinion. Some of the reasons why you would need a second opinion are:

- Your symptoms suggest that you have a non-BPD condition.

- You have suffered a head injury in the past and the doctor wants to rule out any conditions related to your injury.

- Some of your symptoms are related to other medical conditions and must be assessed by a primary care doctor.

It is often challenging to accurately diagnose BPD; therefore, this initial assessment process requires a lot of patience. If you are fortunate to find a good doctor, you will receive a diagnosis immediately after the first assessment and begin your treatment plan soon after. If you are not able to get a good first assessment, be open to approaching different doctors and hearing what they have to say, or how they would treat your symptoms.

Diagnosing BPD

Personality disorders become more apparent during your teenage years. Thus, most diagnoses for BPD occur after you turn 18. This doesn't mean that there aren't any exceptions: In some instances, children under the age of 18 can be diagnosed with BPD if their symptoms are severe and last for more than a year. The risk factors addressed in Chapter 1 make you vulnerable to BPD, however, so do other medical conditions like anxiety, depression, addiction, or eating disorders.

Another important thing to consider when diagnosing BPD is that the condition exists on a spectrum. This means that not every borderline will display the same symptoms or meet the full list of criteria mentioned in the DSM-5. For example, out of the nine criteria listed for BPD, you are only required to exhibit five. If you display symptoms of BPD but don't necessarily meet the criteria, you may need to explore the subtypes of BPD (more about this in the following section).

When assessing your symptoms, medical professionals will consult the DSM-5, a manual published by the APA that offers diagnostic information for universally recognized mental health disorders. For each mental health condition, the DSM-5 highlights a list of symptoms and suggests how many symptoms are mandatory in order to be diagnosed with that particular condition.

The criteria for being diagnosed with BPD is provided below. Generally, a BPD diagnosis would be made if you answered 'yes' to five or more of the following questions (NHS, 2021):

- Do you experience an intense fear when you are left

alone, which causes you to act in inappropriate ways, like constantly calling someone or engaging in self-harming behaviors?

- Would you describe your relationships with others as unstable? Do your feelings toward others switch from being strongly attracted to them (bordering on obsessed) to not trusting them or withdrawing emotionally?

- Are you easily swayed by other people's attitudes and behaviors? Are you confused about who you are?

- Do you often engage in impulsive behaviors, such as abusing drugs and alcohol, reckless spending, or having unsafe sex?

- Have you made repeated suicide attempts in the past or engaged in forms of self-harm?

- Do you often have unexplained mood swings, such as feeling extreme joy one moment and then irritability when a slight change occurs in your environment? Do these mood swings last between a few hours to several days?

- Do you often feel empty inside, as though you are lacking something vital in your life? Are you constantly lonely, even though you have close friends and family?

- Do you have trouble controlling your anger when you are upset? Do you find that you get angry over trivial circumstances (things that other people would normally brush off)?

- When you are in a stressful situation, do you feel distrustful of others or threatened by the world? Do you experience a strong urge to disconnect from others and perform unusual behaviors to protect yourself?

When you finally receive the BPD diagnosis, it is advised to inform close friends and family about it. This is because your BPD symptoms affect your personal and professional relationships. Making them aware of your condition can relieve some of the stress that your relationships are under. How much to disclose about your condition, if anything at all, is completely up to you.

The Subtypes of BPD

In his book, *Disorders of Personality: DSM-IV and Beyond*, psychologist Theodore Millon discovered four subtypes of BPD that are not included in the DSM (Millon & Davis, 1996). These subtypes are:

- Discouraged Borderline Personality Disorder
- Impulsive Borderline Personality Disorder
- Petulant Borderline
- Self-destructive Borderline

People living with BPD may or may not exhibit symptoms of these subtypes, although some individuals may fall under multiple subtypes. Below is an explanation of the four subtypes, showing how each subtype behaves.

The Discouraged Borderline

This individual tends to exhibit signs of dependency in relationships. They cling onto others and are more agreeable with the crowd. Even though a discouraged borderline will seldom spend time alone, they carry a deep sense of sadness. They are often resentful for putting up with other people's bad treatment, but due to their need for others, these feelings cannot be expressed or addressed through meaningful conversation. To cope with their disappointment, the discouraged borderline may turn to harmful coping strategies, like binge drinking or cutting.

When diagnosing discouraged borderline personality disorder, medical professionals tend to look for the following symptoms:

- **Unstable self-image:** Thinking low of yourself, which may lead to self-criticism and stress-induced dissociative states.

- **Decreased empathy:** Showing an inability to understand another person's perspective, while simultaneously being extremely sensitive to perceived criticism or rejection from others.

- **Placing a strong emphasis on loyalty in relationships:** Due to their deep fear of abandonment, they are unwavering when it comes to loyalty. Any signs of mistrust or betrayal may be grounds for terminating the relationship; people are often viewed as being good or bad.

Taylor was diagnosed with a discouraged borderline personality disorder shortly after she became a new mother. To the outside world, it looked like she was enjoying life with her newborn baby and the responsibilities it came with. But that was all an act. Deep down inside she was battling anxiety and thoughts of inadequacy.

Growing up, Taylor was mocked for showing emotions. Her parents would call her weak and tell her to toughen up like her brothers. At school, she was bullied for being soft-spoken. None of her family or teachers found out about this because she learned to internalize her feelings. Instead of lashing out at the bullies or expressing how she felt, she would beat herself up emotionally for being 'weak' and 'embarrassing'.

The harsh self-criticism turned into a violent self-punishment. But, of course, no one could tell how abusive she was being toward herself behind closed doors. She knew how to go from being the life of the party in front of others to the worst tyrant when she was alone.

Fast forward to Taylor as a mother and the inner tyrant had not disappeared. She continued to fight against her thoughts and emotions, hiding what she genuinely felt and showcasing a false self-image. Who would ever know that underneath that display of confidence was an unstable individual who was afraid of ever revealing how scared, insecure, and hypersensitive she really was?

The Impulsive Borderline

An impulsive borderline is a charming and often flirtatious individual who captivates those around them. They may struggle to maintain long-term relationships due to their need for constant validation and their desire to search for the next thrill or adventure. An impulsive borderline will often make decisions without thinking about the consequences of their actions, then later appear remorseful for what they have done. Nonetheless, their charm is usually enough to get them out of trouble— however, it isn't long before they unintentionally create discord in their relationships.

Some of the symptoms unique to impulsive borderline personality disorder include:

- **Exhibiting flirtatious behavior:** Being flirtatious with others, sometimes without realizing it. The impulsive borderline may simply be so fascinated by somebody that it seems like they are attracted to them.

- **Shallow relationships:** Charming personality that is able to draw people near them. However, impulsive people with BPD are not able to sustain relationships beyond the superficial level. Their constant search for thrill causes them to be easily bored or lose interest in others.

- **Reassurance-seeking behaviors:** The need for constant reassurance drives impulsive people with BPD to partake in risky behaviors, complain of recurring illnesses, or act in promiscuous ways to gain attention.

Jared was a hopeless romantic. Well, at least that's what he would tell every unsuspecting victim who found themselves allured by him. He had a knack for getting people to open up about themselves, as though they had known each other for many years. His attraction to an individual would escalate within a matter of weeks. "I like you," would turn into "I love you," then "Let's move in together!"

Neither Jared nor his lovers could see the imminent crash awaiting them. The incredible passion and steamy intimacy would soon be replaced by unanswered texts, silent treatment, and unnecessary arguing. You see, the intensity of the relationship was fun for awhile, but it soon triggered Jared's fear of abandonment. He imagined that the person he loved so much would one day decide to end the relationship, and this caused him a great deal of anxiety and insecurity.

Pushing others away was his way of asking for space to breathe. Although what he didn't realize was that his need for distance felt like rejection. It would come as a shock to him when his lovers would ask for a break up. "How could they do this to me?" he would think, "I trusted them and now my worst fears have come to life!"

But just as quickly as Jared was able to fall in love, he was able to fall out of love. Only a few days would pass before he found his next unsuspecting victim. The cycle of love bombing, showing signs of commitment, then following these with cold and distant behavior would start again.

The Petulant Borderline

A petulant borderline can be described as someone impatient, unpredictable, and extremely irritable. They are often complaining or expressing their negative views about someone or some life event. They can display paranoia and keep their distance from people or uncertain situations, but at the same time, they deeply desire closeness with others. When a petulant borderline gets angry, their reaction can quickly become explosive. Their strong feelings of anger often hide deeper insecurities and resentment.

Some of the striking signs of petulant borderline personality disorder that doctors look for include:

- **Unexplained emotional outbursts:** The petulant borderline's impatience often results in unexpected fits of rage directed at others. This is especially seen when their needs are not met, or when they receive perceived criticism. Due to their emotional outbursts, those around them walk on eggshells and strive to meet their exceedingly high expectations.

- **Passive-aggressive behaviors:** Another indirect way to

41

express anger is through passive-aggressive behaviors, such as being sarcastic, manipulative, or orchestrating subtle acts of sabotage in relationships like 'forgetting' to cook dinner even though that is the household task assigned to you.

- **Push-and-pull patterns in relationships:** Intimacy feels extremely uncomfortable for petulant people with BPD— thus they are likely to push people away with their anger or high expectations. However, when there is too much distance, this can trigger their fear of abandonment and, as a result, they may switch attitudes and shower the same people they pushed away with extreme displays of love.

Brianna's petulant borderline personality disorder was often triggered whenever others challenged her decisions. It could be the smallest thing like asking her to clarify what she had said or disagreeing with her opinion. When people did this, it took her back to her childhood where she was raised by an emotionally abusive father.

In a violent fit of rage, she would have a blackout, and respond to whoever was surrounding her as though she was standing up to her father. The anger unleashed never matched the context of the situation. Her emotions were almost exaggerated, aggressive, and intended to inflict as much pain as possible. Needless to say, in that moment of rage, Brianna would say anything to hurt the other person (sometimes, she wouldn't even remember these words when she had calmed down).

Eventually, she would snap back to reality and regain some sense of normality. Yes, the storm had passed, however she would be the only one left standing after the great amount of destruction caused. Feelings of guilt and embarrassment would sweep over her. "I really messed up this time," she would think to herself, "They will never forgive me." The truth is Brianna was so used to the push-and-pull dynamic in her relationships that every fight would soon be followed by displays of remorse and asking for forgiveness. It wouldn't take long before someone challenged Brianna's decisions again and her fiery rage would be unchained.

The Self-Destructive Borderline

A self-destructive borderline internalizes their deep feelings of shame and resentment and directs their attacks inward. They find conscious or unconscious ways to punish themselves by turning to self-destructive behaviors. What fuels their self-destructive behaviors is self-hatred and a sense of unworthiness. Depending on the severity of their self-hatred, their behaviors can range from drug or alcohol addiction to performing dehumanizing sexual acts.

Some of the symptoms unique to self-destructive borderline personality disorder include:

- **Tendency to self-sabotage:** Due to their intense self-loathing, self-destructive people with BPD often ruin their own chances of success at work and in relationships whenever they seem to be making progress.

- **Unstable sense of self:** They depend on others to validate who they are, and, when faced with criticism, they can become extremely disappointed in themselves, to the extent of self-harming.

- **Deep feelings of resentment:** Tendency to experience mood swings or passive-aggressive behavior as a result of the internalized bitterness they are bottling up. Without acknowledging their pain and repressed desires, it can be

43

difficult to treat these feelings of resentment in therapy.

Tom was diagnosed with self-destructive borderline disorder. This happened shortly after he was diagnosed with compulsive overeating. Since the age of 10 when he was sexually assaulted, he had always had an unhealthy relationship with food. At times, he would use food to numb himself from feeling sad, and other times he would eat in hopes of gaining so much weight that nobody would find him attractive.

According to him, every binge was the last one. There is no doubt that Tom wanted to stop abusing his body with excessive food, but he couldn't resist punishing himself. He blamed the sexual assault for ruining his life and making it difficult to love himself. And since he didn't love himself, it didn't seem possible that anyone else could.

It can be easy to look at any of these four subtypes and discount them as signs of "bad behavior". However, we must remember that these behaviors are signs of mental illness and those suffering with BPD must be treated with respect and compassion. Their unusual, destructive, or attention-seeking behaviors are requests for help and medical treatment.

Chapter Takeaways

Diagnosing BPD can be a drawn out process, especially when your symptoms are not understood. Engaging with the right medical professional who has experience diagnosing and treating BPD (and who is a trained DBT practitioner) will reduce the likelihood of misdiagnosis. During the assessment, the doctor will evaluate your symptoms based on the DSM-5 criteria and see whether you meet the diagnostic requirements for BPD. Since BPD symptoms overlap with symptoms of other medical conditions, it is possible to be diagnosed with a similar condition. Remember, if you or the doctor are not satisfied with the assessment, you are welcome to seek a second or third opinion from another medical doctor.

Besides the four subtypes discovered by Theodore Millon, there is another common subtype known as quiet borderline personality disorder, which is also not included in the DSM-5. We will discuss this subtype in more detail in the following chapter.

CHAPTER 5:

What Is Quiet BPD?

You are so good. So good, you're always feeling so much. And sometimes it feels like you're gonna burst wide open from all the feeling, doesn't it? People like you are the best in the world, but you sure do suffer for it.

- Friedrich Nietzsche

In this chapter you will learn:

- The signs and symptoms of quiet BPD.

- How it differs from traditional BPD.

Acting In vs. Acting Out

BPD is often characterized by intense emotions and unusual or impulsive behaviors directed outward. When these same emotions and behaviors are directed inward, a subtype emerges known as quiet borderline personality disorder.

Similar to the other subtypes, quiet BPD is not recognized in the DSM-5. Someone is usually diagnosed with BPD, then later, upon further evaluation, may receive treatment to address symptoms of quiet BPD. What makes this subtype of BPD difficult to treat is the fact that it is so subtle and barely noticeable in social interactions.

For example, unlike someone with BPD, a person with quiet BPD is capable of maintaining what seems to be 'healthy' relationships. Instead of acting out and projecting their emotions onto others, they internalize everything that they feel and often talk down or punish themselves for the hidden pain and suffering they are carrying.

The symptoms of quiet BPD overlap with symptoms of discouraged BPD and what is known as high-functioning BPD. What all of these subtypes have in common is the inability to communicate thoughts and feelings openly due to the fear of rejection or abandonment. Thus, relationships are often idealized (even when they are dysfunctional or rife with codependency), and the individual deals with their mood swings, irritability, or feelings of emptiness privately.

Identifying the Signs of Quiet BPD

Since quiet BPD is less noticeable than BPD, it is usually misdiagnosed as social anxiety, autism, or depression. When seeking an assessment, it may be useful to approach a doctor who has treated patients with various subtypes of BPD, who didn't necessarily exhibit explosive emotions or struggled to maintain their jobs or relationships.

Below are some of the signs that are unique to quiet BPD, which can assist you in getting the right diagnosis:

1. Regular Mood Swings

You frequently feel emotionally unstable, or are triggered by the slightest changes in your environment. Instead of acting out what you are feeling, you sit with those intense emotions in silence, showing very little signs of emotional distress. You may even emotionally shut down, as a defense mechanism, when faced with severe challenges.

2. People-Pleasing

It is hard for you to set healthy boundaries with others because that would mean opening up and expressing how you feel. Instead of being open and transparent with others, you will likely turn a blind eye to unacceptable behaviors, walk on eggshells around temperamental people, or make excuses for bad behavior.

3. Blaming Yourself

A fear of rejection and abandonment makes it difficult to hold others accountable for their actions. When you are feeling frustrated, you tend to direct that frustration inward and blame yourself for tolerating abuse, not standing up for yourself, or any rising conflict within your relationships. You erroneously think that if you behaved differently, the chaos erupting in your life wouldn't happen.

4. Fear of Emotional Intimacy

Living with quiet BPD, similar to any other subtype of BPD, causes you to feel afraid of others coming too close, particularly to the extent that they might see who you really are. For as long as you can wear the mask and pretend to be calm, cool, and collected, you can enjoy surface-level relationships. The thought of someone getting so close to you and potentially leaving you or hurting you is unbearable. You also might think that if someone discovered how emotionally volatile you are, they would be repulsed and walk away from you.

5. Suppressing Emotions

Due to your childhood upbringing—what you saw, learned, and experienced—you tend to hide your emotions. Perhaps you grew up in a household where it wasn't safe to express your thoughts and feelings, and, as an adult, you find that relationships are less stressful when you keep your true thoughts and feelings to yourself. Over the years, you have learned to only display emotions that are positive and cater to the needs of others, while hiding negative emotions and sentiments that would cause conflict.

All of these signs or symptoms reinforce a sense of separateness or isolation from others. A deeper part of you has always felt disconnected from others (even from your own life to some extent), but when you find it difficult to embrace who you are and allow others in, you can feel like you are living a double life.

Under-Control vs. Over-Control

There are various forms of therapy that can treat BPD, but typically when you are diagnosed with quiet BPD, those interventions may not be as successful. For example, instead of practicing DBT, you may benefit from radically open dialectical behavior therapy (RO-DBT).

One of the reasons why quiet people with BPD require a slightly different intervention is because they have issues with being over-controlled and highly functional, rather than under-controlled and dysregulated. The over-control/under-control construct was discovered by Dr. Thomas Lynch and his colleagues. This was after they realized that some BPD patients were not responding well to DBT. These patients tended to display signs of being over-controlled and having a high tolerance for emotional distress.

Nevertheless, this didn't mean that they felt nothing. In fact, patients who were over-controlled experienced the same kind of sensitivity to threats as any other BPD patient, but they would hide their emotions and appear aloof.

Lynch believed that BPD patients classified as over-controlled exhibited the following deficits:

- **Lack of openness and reciprocity:** Tendency to be dismissive of other people's feedback or opinions, as well as being risk-averse or suspicious of novel experiences.

- **Lack of spontaneity or flexibility:** Desiring to be in control of routines, plans, and schedules, to the extent of creating a predictable environment. Life is experienced through a set of conscious or unconscious rules that serve as the standard of behavior expected from yourself and others.

- **Lack of emotional awareness:** Tendency to feel uncomfortable expressing emotions spontaneously or responding to another person's emotional outburst. You may desire to contain emotions or focus on deciding when feeling a certain way is acceptable or unacceptable.

- **Lack of social connectedness:** Finding it difficult to open up to others, engage freely in unstructured conversations, or share how you feel. Closeness and intimacy could trigger you to push others away or emotionally shut down.

In relationships, being over-controlled may appear as avoidant attachment, or keeping people at arm's length. However, deep down, you may desire closeness but fear that others will take advantage of your vulnerability. As a child, you may have internalized the message that showing emotions or opening yourself to others leads to heartache, rejection, or neglect. Therefore, as a measure to protect yourself, you learned how to be extremely self-reliant and accumulate power, wealth, and knowledge to feel safe.

Kate suffered from quiet BPD, which meant that when her stress levels were high, she became strangely calm. Appearing aloof and emotionally flat was her way of managing anxiety and somehow gaining control of the threatening situation she was placed under. In group settings, she would speak in clichés or offer generic statements—any kind of surface-level conversation that wouldn't make her feel more vulnerable than she already did.

Due to her lack of emotional awareness, Kate's relationships took a heavy blow. Her friends cited that she seemed spaced out most of the time. One friend even mentioned that she couldn't tell what Kate needed or how to support her. Not once did Kate take the opportunity to explain her condition. Her fear of suffering more rejection subdued her into silence. Instead, she would sulk and become withdrawn from her friends (a condition known as splitting), until she was ready to socialize again.

Chapter Takeaways

What makes quiet BPD different from traditional BPD is the fact that the symptoms are hidden. It can be difficult to identify someone with quiet BPD because they are highly functional and are capable of maintaining work and personal relationships. Due to the sense of shame they feel about their own emotional experiences, they are also less likely to seek treatment or open up to others about what they are going through. Some of the tell-tale signs that someone may be suffering with quiet BPD are them being overly independent, appearing aloof or unfeeling, being a people-pleaser, avoiding conflict or controversy, and having more shallow or surface-level relationships than close ones.

Once you have understood your diagnosis and its potential subtypes, it is time to explore the variety of treatments available to you.

PART 2:

Exploring BPD

Treatment Options

CHAPTER 6:

Dialectical Behavior Therapy

I still get very high and very low in life. Daily. But I've finally accepted the fact that being sensitive is just how I was made, that I don't have to hide it and I don't have to fix it. I'm not broken.

- Glennon Doyle Melton

In this chapter you will learn:

- About the structure of DBT and what to expect at your therapy sessions.

- What the four main DBT skills are, as well as exercises to practice at home.

How Does DBT Work?

You received a brief introduction to DBT in Chapter 2; in this chapter, we are going to take a closer look at this popular treatment and the ways it can address BPD symptoms.

Dialectical behavior therapy (DBT) is a type of cognitive

behavior therapy (CBT) that is focused on helping people adapt to difficult life circumstances (Buffum Taylor, 2022). It does this through championing two opposing ideas: accepting the reality of life, and changing harmful behaviors. The major difference between DBT and CBT is that the former teaches people how to cope with and accept intense emotions, rather than seeking to get rid of them, while the latter seeks to regulate or replace harmful thoughts and emotions.

DBT is administered by a certified DBT therapist who can be a psychologist, psychiatrist, family therapist, or social worker. Finding the right therapist can be a lengthy process, especially when you are searching for someone with experience treating BPD and similar mental disorders. It is the DBT therapist's job to help you learn to accept your mental health condition and actively seek to change harmful behaviors by learning healthy coping skills. After attending some sessions, you will have the tools to continue building your DBT skills sets at home.

Originally, DBT was designed for high-risk patients suffering from suicidal thoughts and BPD. The creator, Dr. Marsha Linehan, ran an experiment on patients who were hospitalized for suicidal behaviors. The success of her trial, and many other similar trials, caused doctors to prescribe DBT when treating other mental health disorders too.

DBT is one of the treatments for BPD that is endorsed by the APA, and it has been found to be effective in treating the following symptoms:

- Reducing suicidal behaviors
- Shortening hospital stays
- Minimizing emotional outbursts

- Reducing the likelihood of the patient abandoning treatment

- Improved social skills

DBT is a structured form of therapy that addresses multiple symptoms of BPD in stages. The first stage is to root out self-destructive behaviors, like self-harming or suicidal thoughts and attempts. Once that has been addressed, the therapist will move to the second stage and teach you skills to improve your quality of life, such as emotional regulation, self-awareness, and coping with change. The third stage focuses on improving the quality of your relationships, as well as your self-image. Then, finally, the therapist will help you plan major lifestyle changes, like replacing harmful habits, finding meaningful work and relationships, and picking up healthy hobbies and interests.

The Four DBT Skills

During your DBT sessions, you will learn how to apply four skills, also known as modules, in your life. The purpose of these skills is to help you find productive ways of dealing with intense emotions and challenging life situations. Below is an in-depth look at each skill and a few exercises that you can practice at home!

Mindfulness

Mindfulness is the practice of paying attention to what is happening in the present moment, observing your thoughts, and accepting whatever feelings may arise. Mindfulness skills get you to the point of accepting who you are, how you experience life, and adapting to situations that you cannot control.

One of the ways to become more mindful is to tap into the "wise mind". In DBT, the mind is understood as having three states: emotional, rational, and wise. Each state of mind can be useful, depending on when and how it is used—however, the wise mind is the ultimate state of mind that creates a balance between emotional and rational thinking.

It is common for people with BPD to be trapped in an emotional state of mind, where life events are interpreted based on feeling. As a result, emotions are confused as facts, and this can distort reality. Examples of behaviors influenced by the emotional mind include:

- Losing your temper at a store manager because they don't have a product in stock.

- Going out clubbing every weekend because it is fun.

- Making an impulsive decision, like traveling to a nearby city.

- Purchasing an item that you cannot afford.

- Seeing someone that you disagree with (or who disagrees with you) as an enemy.

The rational mind favors logic and reasoning over emotions. It interprets the world based on learned patterns, beliefs, and common sense. A quiet borderline is more likely to rely on their rational mind to navigate through life, out of fear of being led by emotion. Nevertheless, too much rational mind leads to rigidity, risk-aversion, and the inability to adapt to unexpected life situations. Examples of behaviors influenced by the rational mind include:

- Living a structured and planned life.

- Making decisions based on outcomes from past experiences.

- Evaluating the cause and effect of taking action.

- Interpreting people's behaviors at face value; seeing people as one-dimensional.

Since people with BPD tend to experience life in extremes, it is important for them to learn how to balance emotions with logic. The wise state of mind is where the emotional and rational overlap, creating a more grounded and neutral experience of reality. According to Dr. Linehan, everyone has a wise mind, even though sometimes it can be difficult to trace. Through practicing mindfulness skills and exercises like meditation, you can locate your wise mind and discover the following:

- A sense of calm in your mind *and* body.

- Feeling as though you are observing the unfolding of a situation, rather than actively participating in it.

- Intuitively knowing the right thing to do.

- A sense of relief following a challenging situation; knowing deep down that everything is going to be okay.

- Seeing a situation through a wider lens; taking into consideration the full picture, instead of segments.

Mindfulness Exercise

Schedule five minute rest breaks throughout your day. During the five minutes, put down all your electronics, close your eyes, and sit back in a comfortable position. In your head, ask yourself how you are doing, then listen for whatever thoughts or emotions arise. As your thoughts and emotions present themselves, treat each one with compassion and look at what they are pointing at. Don't judge them for being right or wrong, appropriate or inappropriate; simply create a loving space for them to be seen and embraced.

After the five minutes is complete, write down what thoughts or emotions came up in a notebook. Every evening, before you go to bed, look at the notes for the day and notice any patterns of thinking that emerge. Do these patterns show that you are mostly engaging your emotional, rational, or wise mind? What new information are you learning about yourself?

Distress Tolerance

Mindfulness skills teach you how to be in the moment and acknowledge your thoughts and emotions. However, in a crisis, these skills are not enough. You need a different set of skills that can help you remain resilient during tough times and prevent you from turning to destructive behaviors.

Think of distress tolerance skills as the survival skills that offer you practical ways to cope with intense emotions, unexpected life events, and intrusive thoughts. Whenever you feel as though you want to fight, withdraw from others, or tense up, these skills can reduce stress and anxiety, and help you overcome the situation.

Some of the many benefits of distress tolerance skills are:

- Helping you face challenges head on, rather than walking away.

- Improving the belief you have within yourself to overcome difficulties.

- Weighing the pros and cons of different coping strategies before choosing the appropriate response.

- Finding ways to self-soothe and calm emotional triggers.

One of the popular distress tolerance skills taught is known as **Wise Mind A.C.C.E.P.T.S.** It provides action steps (**A.C.C.E.P.T.S.**) that you can practice whenever you seek to distract yourself from intense emotions (DBT Self-Help, n.d.). When practicing these steps, remember to switch to your wise mind—the state of mind that feels balanced and intuitive. Below is a breakdown of each action step:

A—Activities: Create a list of activities that you can shift your focus to whenever you are stressed. These can include activities that help you relax, engage your creative brain, or make you feel good about yourself. Have this list available in digital and printed format, so that during a moment of intense panic, you can turn to the list quickly.

C—Contributing: Focus on someone or something else that is unrelated to your current situation. It could be calling a close friend and checking up on them, volunteering at a local animal shelter, writing a letter of gratitude to a coworker who has been helpful recently, etc. Helping others will reduce your feelings of distress, improve your mood, and help you view your troubling situation within the broader context of life.

C—Comparisons: Take 10–15 minutes to reflect on the person you used to be 10–15 years ago. Think back to the kinds of life situations you were dealing with and how you managed to cope. This exercise is mostly effective when you compare your current life situation to a time in the past when you didn't cope as well. The purpose of doing this is to help you recognize that, compared to the past, you are in a much more favorable position and you have the strength to overcome this obstacle too.

E—Emotions: Another way to distract yourself from intense emotions is to cultivate a positive one. Remember, your mind decides which emotion is most suitable in each situation. If you tend to react with anger, then it means that in the past anger was seen to be the most suitable way to convey what you were feeling. But you don't have to remain loyal to anger if it no longer serves you. One of the ways to cultivate positive emotions during stressful situations is to turn to activities that trigger positive feelings, such as listening to a guided meditation, watching stand-up comedy, playing with your pets, or writing in your journal.

P—Pushing away: You have the power to choose what you focus your attention on. As soon as your attention shifts from one object or thought to another, the level of interest fades too. When you are in a stressful situation, shift your attention away from the situation or thought to something more desirable. This could mean walking away from the violent person or triggering environment and finding a safe place to spend some time alone. If the pain is caused by internal thoughts, close your eyes and visualize that you have filled a box with everything that is troubling you and placed the box in a closet. Reassure yourself that you will process the pain later on when you are feeling stronger.

T—Thoughts: What often worsens feelings of distress is overthinking. Your mind goes on overdrive and attempts to come up with multiple options and scenarios to best handle the situation. You can distract your mind by engaging in mental activities that relieve anxious thoughts, such as doing a crossword puzzle, reading a book, or creating a task list. These mental activities are meant to delay the urge to turn to self-destructive behaviors while your stress levels decrease.

S—Sensations: By engaging your five senses—sight, smell, touch, taste, and hearing—you can find positive ways to self-soothe. This is also known as 'grounding'. When you are grounded, your mind is focused on what it can perceive through the senses, rather than what it imagines.

Below are a few ideas on ways that you can activate your senses (Salters-Pedneault, 2020):

- Sing along to your favorite song.
- Read a piece of poetry, or a chapter from a book.
- Call a loved one.
- Write down a few mantras, like "I am wanted," or "I am safe," to reduce whatever intense emotion you may be feeling. Repeat the mantra until you feel grounded.
- Watch a funny video on YouTube or an episode of your favorite TV sitcom.
- Download an app that offers you a selection of nature sounds. Whenever you are feeling distressed, play a sound and focus on slowing down your breathing.
- Take a dip in a swimming pool or have a cool shower. You can also run your hands under cold tap water or take a hot bubble bath.
- Take a rubber band and gently snap it on your wrist.
- After a shower, massage scented lotion or oil on your body and focus on the way it feels and smells as you work it into your skin.

Interpersonal Effectiveness

Both quiet and traditional people with BPD experience difficulty expressing their needs appropriately. The quiet borderline may pretend as though they don't have needs, while the traditional borderline may react disproportionately when their needs are not met. Interpersonal effectiveness skills are centered around strengthening relationships through open, clear, and compassionate communication. They teach you how to resolve conflict, set healthy boundaries, and express needs and desires effectively, without hurting another person.

A popular interpersonal effectiveness skill taught in DBT is **D.E.A.R. M.A.N.** It offers you action steps on how to make requests or engage in tough conversations with others. The aim is to clearly communicate what you need without being either forceful or passive. Even though there is no guarantee that the other person will listen to you, this skill can reduce misunderstandings and increase the confidence you have within yourself. Below is a guideline on how to use **D.E.A.R. M.A.N.**:

D—Describe: Using clear and direct language, describe the situation at hand to the other person. If your feelings were hurt, give them context about what happened that might have offended you. Avoid making any judgments or speaking in a threatening or condescending tone. The purpose of describing the situation is to help the other person see where you are coming from, and how both of you can find a solution together.

E—Express: In the simplest way, express how the situation has made you feel. Begin your sentences with "I feel" as a way to show ownership of your emotional experience and avoid passing blame. You don't have to go into great detail about your feelings; what's important is that you share the emotional impact.

A—Assert: State what you need to take place so you can both move forward peaceably. Try not to overthink the solution or water it down because you are afraid of how it will be received.

The more comfortable you become asserting your needs, the easier it will be to set healthy boundaries and feel safe in your relationships going forward.

R—Reinforce: Be clear about the payoff for having your needs met. For instance, will it make you feel respected? Will you feel a deeper sense of appreciation for the other person? If you are drawing a boundary, reinforce the negative consequence that will follow if the boundary is violated again. For instance, will you stop making time to see the other person? Or will you stop inviting them to your house?

M—Be mindful: During the conversation, it can be easy to forget the main objective for having the discussion. This is particularly true when you are speaking to someone who may be manipulative and try to spin the truth or deflect. Don't hesitate to take a few moments to breathe, recollect yourself, and be mindful of your objectives. Ask yourself if you are closer or farther away from achieving the objectives of the discussion. Remember, you cannot control the other person's responses or behaviors, but you can ensure that you have brought forward your thoughts and feelings in a clear and respectful way.

A—Appear confident: When getting your points across, pay attention to your body language, tone of voice, and facial expressions. These are all non-verbal cues that project confidence or a lack of it. When you seem like you are unsure of yourself, the other person may find it difficult to take your requests seriously. Therefore, present yourself as someone who knows what they want and has enough courage to ask for it. The great thing about confidence is that you don't have to have it to appear as though you do. Practice looking into a mirror and speaking like somebody whose confidence you admire. Who knows? Eventually, your confidence may start to come naturally.

N—Negotiate: One of the skills that can be difficult for people with BPD is compromising. When a person with BPD has their mind set on something, they can feel a sense of rejection when their request isn't fulfilled accordingly. However, human beings are not robots that all think, feel, and make decisions alike. Each individual has a unique perspective on life and what they believe should be done in any given situation. Be flexible enough to make compromises or find a middle ground, so that the end result is an outcome that both you and the other person are proud of. Think in terms of reaching a win-win situation, where both parties have to make sacrifices to reach a mutual agreement, but both parties ultimately benefit as well.

If you sense that you are getting heated up during the D.E.A.R. M.A.N. conversation, excuse yourself and take a few minutes to calm down. The purpose of the conversation is to talk about difficult matters in a way that strengthens your relationship.

Below is an example of how the D.E.A.R. M.A.N conversation would sound if you wanted to renegotiate who cooks dinner at home:

Describe: I am the only person in the house who cooks dinner. Sometimes, I return from work tired and have to push myself to prepare a meal for everyone.

Express: I feel frustrated that nobody will share this responsibility with me. I feel like my need for rest is not being considered.

Assert: I am not willing to continue like this. I need you to share the responsibility of cooking with me. Perhaps we can decide on days that suit each of us better.

Reinforce: By helping me with this task, you will take a huge load off my shoulders. Coming home won't feel as stressful as it does right now.

Be mindful: [Repeat the objective of this discussion and reinforce the desired positive outcomes.]

Appear confident: [Maintain eye contact, loosen your face muscles and offer reassuring smiles; speak in an assertive but compassionate tone of voice.]

Negotiate: I am happy to cook on Mondays and Tuesdays because I know you usually leave work late on those days. I can also cook on one day of the weekend.

Emotion Regulation

It is common for a person with BPD to feel as though they cannot escape experiencing intense emotions or having strong reactions to everyday challenges. The aim of emotion regulation skills is not to minimize the emotional impact that you might go through when feeling triggered, but instead to make it easier to cope and endure through those intense moments. If possible, emotion regulation skills can also be used as part of your crisis management plan. When you sense strong emotions welling up inside, you can turn to one of the skills to prevent further emotional distress.

Some of the benefits of learning emotion regulation skills are:

- An increased ability to recognize and label different emotions.

- Reduced feelings of vulnerability when identifying and sharing emotions.

- Learning how to be mindful of emotions without judging them as good or bad.

- An increased ability to control emotional impulses.

A core emotion regulation skill is learning how to identify and describe emotions. This is important because it gives you a greater sense of control over your emotional experience. Knowing what you are feeling can quickly point you to the 'why' and help you associate an emotion with a life event taking place. By managing your emotions, you are also able to manage your thoughts and behaviors, which means that you are less likely to overreact (or at least you will be more aware of your overreactions). The following steps are useful in identifying and describing emotions:

1. Identify the Prompting Event

Emotions can be triggered by external factors, such as being in the company of certain people, watching a TV show, scrolling through social media, or being in a specific environment. The best way to identify a prompting event is to get into the habit of writing down what took place moments before you felt triggered. Soon enough, you will start to identify patterns of situations that frequently trigger you.

2. Get Behind the Interpretation

In most cases, emotions arise due to how you interpret an experience. If you believe that you are under threat, you will respond with fear or anxiety, whereas if you believe you are being criticized, you will respond with anger. Learn to pause for a moment and reflect on how you interpret a situation unfolding right before you. Ask yourself, "What do I think is happening right now?" or "How do I feel I am being impacted by this situation?" The same situation can trigger different kinds of emotions, depending on your interpretation. This means that you can also change your emotional response by perceiving the situation differently.

3. Tune Into Your Body

The mind-body connection is a fascinating phenomenon. It explains how thoughts and emotions become physical manifestations in the body. For instance, your anxious thoughts can lead to an increased heart rate, sweaty palms, or stomach cramps. Learning how to tune into your physical sensations can help you identify emotions. Of course, this isn't easy, especially if you are disconnected from your body.

It might take practice to associate a specific body sensation with an emotion, but this can be achieved through journaling. All it takes is being mindful and noticing the moment-by-moment changes you are feeling. For example, you can notice how your breathing rate changes when you step outside of the house, or how your face muscles tighten when you are speaking to strangers. Write down all of these observations, as they will unconsciously communicate what you are feeling in that moment.

4. Notice the Urges

Each individual reacts differently to emotions. For one person, anger might make them yell, whereas for another person, anger might make them retreat in silence. Nevertheless, all emotions prompt some kind of behavior, and it can be useful to identify what urges you feel whenever you are triggered by various emotions.

Noticing your urges can be empowering because it puts the power back into your own hands. You can choose to notice an urge and not follow through with its promptings. For example, when you are disappointed, there might be a strong urge to abandon your goal or project and walk away. But it is not necessary for you to follow through with this urge. You can choose to carry out different behaviors, like going into problem-solving mode or asking for help.

5. Name Your Emotions

If you are not familiar with paying attention to how you feel, it can be difficult naming your emotions. On the surface, anger, envy, and irritability might feel the same, even though they are three different types of emotions. However, the benefit of learning how to name your emotions is that it can help you understand the emotional impact of every unique life experience.

When naming emotions, the first step is to learn the difference between primary and secondary emotions. Primary emotions are the basic structure that all other emotions are built upon. If you think deeply about how you are feeling, at the root will be a primary emotion. There are six recognized primary emotions:

- Anger

- Fear

- Happiness

- Love

- Joy

- Disgust

For each of these emotions, there are multiple secondary emotions that offer different expressions. For example, anger can be expressed as hurt, being distant, jealousy, or irritation. It is possible to feel angry, then, after some time feel hurt, which in turn causes you to become distant. The ability to trace the chain of your emotions and figure out which emotion led to the next can help you explain your emotional experience.

Refer to the table below to explore the various primary and secondary emotions:

Primary Emotions	Secondary Emotions
Anger	Critical
	Feeling let down
	Provoked
	Bitter
	Irritated
	Disrespected
Fear	Insecure
	Rejected
	Anxious
	Scared
	Vulnerable
	Overwhelmed
	Peaceful

Happiness	Content
	Accepted
	Playful
	Optimistic
	Proud
Love	Compassion
	Attraction
	Passionate
	Lust
	Kindness
	Affection
Joy	Cheerfulness
	Relief
	Hopeful
	Excitement

	Pleasure
	Openness
Disgust	Disappointed
	Judgmental
	Humiliated
	Nauseated
	Loathing
	Disapproving/Unacceptable

Emotion Regulation Exercise

Think about a recent situation that made you emotional. On a piece of paper, answer the following questions:

- What was the prompting event?

- How did you interpret the experience?

- What body sensations confirmed your emotional experience?

- What kind of urges were you compelled to follow?

- Can you describe the chain of emotions, starting with the original primary emotion?

Chapter Takeaways

The reason why DBT is such a popular treatment for BPD is because it emphasizes both acceptance and change. An individual living with BPD is already ashamed of their unexplained or seemingly uncontrollable outbursts or reactions—thus embracing who they are and how differently they respond to life situations can make the treatment process more effective. The four DBT skills provide a practical way for people with BPD to learn how to endure through challenging situations and slowly unlearn harmful coping strategies.

In the following chapter, we will look at other complementary therapies that can be administered alongside DBT.

CHAPTER 7:

Complementary Therapies to Treat BPD

Living with BPD is pure confusion. It's always like: "Am I allowed to be upset about this thing or am I being oversensitive?"

- HealthyPlace

In this chapter you will learn:

- About alternative therapies that are effective in treating BPD.

Cognitive Behavior Therapy (CBT)

The inspiration for DBT came from CBT, a form of psychotherapy that was developed in the 1960s by Dr. Aaron T. Beck (Miller, 2019). CBT was designed to show people how their personal problems are closely related to their quality of thoughts, emotions, and behaviors. Essentially, we are all responsible for our cognitive processes, how we interpret the information we extract from experiences. CBT analyzes those cognitive processes and assesses how helpful or harmful they can be to our mental and emotional well-being.

Similar to DBT, a certified CBT therapist will administer the treatment. However, after some time, you will be equipped with the necessary tools to continue treatment at home. Some of the skills therapists will teach include how to interrupt intrusive thoughts, how to break down problems into smaller chunks of information, and how to replace harmful beliefs with more productive ones.

The key difference in CBT and DBT is the emphasis on validation and relationships. CBT teaches you how to reduce the prevalence of negative thoughts, while DBT teaches you how to embrace them and stop them from getting in the way of your progress. CBT is also more focused on your unique experience of reality, whereas DBT looks at how your thoughts, emotions, and behaviors affect your work and relationships.

One of the goals of CBT is to correct negative thinking, or cognitive distortions. Cognitive distortions are misguided thinking patterns that create problems or trigger real and imagined fears. Together with your therapist, you are invited to explore how your misguided thinking patterns reinforce certain emotions and behaviors. With deeper understanding into the mechanics of your thinking, you are able to adjust and reframe your thoughts to initiate more positive reactions.

There are a multitude of different types of cognitive distortions, and, during therapy, you and your therapist will discover many of them. Below is an example of what cognitive distortions tend to sound like:

- **Overgeneralization:** "I don't deserve to be loved."

- **Moral imperatives:** "*I should* be more caring toward others."

- **Jumping to conclusions:** "My spouse hasn't texted me today. I guess I did something wrong."

- **Mind reading:** "I can tell by her tone that she doesn't like me."

- **Emotional reasoning:** "I felt uncomfortable around him. I doubt he is being truthful."

There are different strategies used in CBT to challenge and correct cognitive distortions, such as increasing self-awareness by recognizing misguided thoughts, identifying thoughts that lead to emotional triggers, and asking yourself reflective questions about your thoughts, such as:

- Is this thought based on facts, or is it an assumption?

- Does this thought reflect what is likely to happen, or is it based on the worst-case scenario?

- Is there any concrete evidence for or against this thought?

- Could there be another way of interpreting the situation?

- Is this thought black-or-white? Could there be a gray area that is being overlooked?

The combination of assessing cognitive processes and seeing what kind of emotions and behaviors they produce is effective in introducing improved coping strategies to encourage positive thinking patterns and productive behaviors.

Mentalization-Based Therapy (MBT)

MBT is a treatment designed for people living with BPD which focuses on understanding cognitive processes, such as how beliefs influence your mental state (Madeson, 2022). The foundation of this therapy is based on the concept of mentalizing, which is the ability to distinguish between what you think and feel and what someone else thinks and feels. Doing this can help you take ownership of your mental and emotional experiences and improve emotional regulation.

There are some similarities between DBT, CBT, and MBT. After all, both DBT and MBT have their roots in CBT. However, there are a few striking differences between MBT and DBT. First, therapists who are trained to administer MBT don't require as much training as those who administer DBT because it is more of a "talk therapy" than a skills-based therapy. Another difference is seen in the treatment goals. The goal of MBT is to strengthen mentalization, whereas in DBT, the goal is to teach acceptance and how to make necessary life changes.

The relationship between the patient and therapist is crucial in order for this treatment to be effective. Most of the time, patients who are drawn to this form of therapy are struggling with trust issues, paranoia, and emotional dysregulation. Therefore, the therapist must create a comfortable environment where the patient feels safe to explore their thoughts and feelings. It is common for levels of mentalizing and emotional arousal to fluctuate during each session.

This is not always a bad thing because some level of responsiveness is required to go deeper into the mind and explore alternative thoughts. However, the therapist will monitor the patient's state of mind and their ability to continue mentalizing when faced with stressful life events like unexpected failure or rejection. The ultimate goal of the therapist is to help the patient learn how to have a balanced perspective on life situations and respond to challenges with appropriate social behaviors.

Transference-Focused Psychotherapy (TFP)

Some of the common issues that people with BPD experience are emotional dysregulation, an unstable sense of self, and troublesome relationships with others. TFP seeks to address these issues by focusing on the relationship between the patient and therapist. The term 'transference' refers to the attitude a patient has toward their therapist. This attitude is typically informed by their attitude toward relationships in the real world.

Similar to traditional talk therapy, the patient and therapist will explore how past experiences influence the patient's current life circumstances. The goal of having these discussions is to help the patient reintegrate their split selves into the broader understanding of who they are. 'Splitting' is a common defense mechanism in people with BPD, where they see something or someone as being all good or all bad, including themselves. They may have trouble seeing themselves as a complex, multi-dimensional person due to this "all-or-nothing" mentality, and it can take speaking to a therapist to strengthen the patient's sense of self and outlook on life.

Research has shown that TFP is effective in treating patients with BPD (McLean Hospital, 2022). In a study published in the Journal of Personality Disorders, BPD patients who were offered TFP treatment for 12 months showed a decrease in suicide attempts, self-harming behaviors, and hospitalization (Clarkin et al., 2001). Another study compared the effectiveness of TFP to other therapies, like DBT and dynamic supportive treatment. The results of the study showed that all three therapies were effective in treating anxiety, depression, and interpersonal effectiveness, but only TFP led to an improvement in verbal attacks and irritability (Clarkin et al., 2007).

What makes TFP unique from other types of psychotherapy is the treatment agreement. Before the treatment program begins, the therapist will enter into an agreement with the patient about the expectations that both parties will need to fulfill. Some of these expectations might include:

- The length of sessions.

- How suicidal feelings will be addressed during sessions (for example, the therapist may request that the patient go to a psychiatric emergency room).

- How and when to contact the therapist outside of the therapy sessions.

As part of the treatment agreement, the therapist will also ask the patient to complete an activity. For instance, they might ask the patient to work, volunteer, or attend school for a minimum of 20 hours per week. This activity is designed to allow the patient to step outside of their comfort zone and engage with the real world. The activity will also offer them plenty of opportunities to interact with different people, and this may bring up personal issues that the patient can talk to the therapist about in their next session.

Over the course of the treatment, the patient's attitude toward the therapist and their environment becomes more trusting and stable. They may come to have a balanced perception of people and of themselves, which allows them to show greater resilience in the face of challenges.

Schema Therapy

Schema therapy is a treatment that combines aspects of CBT, psychoanalysis, and attachment theory. The purpose of the therapy is to help the patient discover their schemas, the harmful patterns that are learned during early childhood when a child's emotional needs aren't met.

As we know, one of the risk factors for BPD is trauma, abuse, or abandonment during childhood. These painful experiences often cause the child to develop maladaptive coping mechanisms, or 'schemas', in response to the perceived threats in their environment. When these schemas are not addressed early on through psychotherapy, they are integrated as part of the self and influence how the person with BPD interacts with the world.

Schema therapy not only exposes these maladaptive coping mechanisms, but also addresses attachment issues that may have been experienced in the parent-child relationship. The therapist will explore the patient's family upbringing and assess which emotional needs were never fulfilled. Some of the core emotional needs required to build a stable sense of self are:

- A sense of safety in relationships.
- Having a strong sense of self-identity.
- Being free to express your thoughts and emotions without fearing judgment or punishment.
- Feeling open enough to play, let loose, and be spontaneous.
- Creating and maintaining healthy boundaries.

The reactions that a patient has to their schemas are known as "coping styles". In other words, when the feeling of rejection arises, the patient might think specific thoughts or carry out specific behaviors. Coping styles are usually as old as the schema itself, and, in most cases, these thoughts and behaviors were once seen as a useful way to avoid pain or difficult emotions. Each patient's coping styles will look different, depending on their personality and what has worked well for them in the past. It is also possible for coping styles to evolve over time, even though the schema stays the same.

The three common coping styles seen in patients are similar to the fight-flight-freeze response. These include:

- **Surrender:** Recognizing the schema and giving into it. This often leads to behaviors that reinforce the schema and make it difficult for you to break destructive patterns.

- **Avoidance:** Recognizing the schema but doing everything in your power to not trigger it. This could mean avoiding being around certain people or situations. This strategy often makes you more vulnerable to behaviors that offer a distraction, such as substance abuse or compulsive behaviors.

- **Overcompensation:** Recognizing the schema and declaring war against it by attempting to display the opposite actions and behaviors. In the short-term, this may offer some relief and feel as though you have overcome the pattern, but in the long-term it tends to lead to rigid, aggressive, controlling, or excessive behaviors.

Together with the therapist, the patient learns how to identify and heal their schemas, adopt healthier coping styles, learn how to reparent themselves by responding to their emotional needs, and find better ways of coping with distress when their needs cannot be met.

Radically Open Dialectical Behavior Therapy (RO-DBT)

RO-DBT is a fairly new treatment that was developed in the early 2000s by psychologist Dr. Thomas R. Lynch (Hempel, 2019). It is based on DBT, but focuses on treating borderline patients who suffer from overcontrol (a symptom that comes with quiet BPD).

As discussed in Chapter 5, the symptoms of quiet BPD are more subtle than traditional BPD. People with quiet BPD have an excessive need for self-control, to the extent that they often live rigid lifestyles, set really high standards for themselves, and will only display behaviors they deem socially acceptable. People with quiet BPD also tend to be self-sacrificing due to their need to please others and avoid conflict. As a result of this, their needs in relationships are often not communicated or responded to.

RO-DBT seeks to treat overcontrol by encouraging radical openness. There are three components to radical openness, which include:

- **Acknowledging stimuli that are felt in the moment:** Showing a willingness to sit with difficult emotions as they arise, acknowledging the impact of certain actions that have been taken, and exploring areas of your life that you seek to avoid.

- **Looking for answers within:** Instead of brushing unwanted emotions off or pretending that you are unaffected by stressful situations, RO-DBT encourages self-inquiry in order to seek understanding about your life experiences, ask tough reflective questions, and be willing to admit when you took the wrong action.

- **Having a more flexible approach to life:** When you

understand that your environment is constantly changing, to reduce feelings of distress, you must be willing to adapt to your current life circumstances. This requires honesty about what reactions or behaviors are no longer effective in maintaining healthy relationships, protecting your boundaries, and having a positive sense of self.

Similar to DBT, this treatment seeks to transfer coping skills that can improve the way people with quiet BPD navigate work and relationships. The four main DBT skills are touched upon during RO-DBT treatment—however, a novel skill that is also taught is "social signaling". Research has shown that people with BPD suffering with overcontrol have a heightened sense of sensitivity that makes it harder for them to feel safe in relationships. Social signaling teaches non-verbal communication strategies to make it easier to express emotions in an appropriate manner.

The theme of radical openness is also not lost throughout the treatment process. Unlike DBT's call for acceptance—which encourages patients to embrace reality—radical openness skills encourage patients to challenge their biases, preconceived ideas, and habitual responses to reality. This is done so that the patient can overcome the mental blocks that cause them to avoid expressing themselves openly.

Chapter Takeaways

As you may have noticed while reading this chapter, there are many different types of therapeutic interventions available for treating BPD. This is a step in the right direction, as more researchers are learning about the symptoms of the disorder and various ways to respond to them. While DBT is heralded as one of the most effective treatments for BPD, it is certainly not the only option. Combining different therapies or hopping from one therapy to the next is common among BPD patients. What's important is finding the right therapies that you can commit to for an extended period of time.

Like any other mental health condition, BPD can be treated with prescription medication. The next chapter will explore the kinds of medication that BPD symptoms respond well to.

CHAPTER 8:

Finding the Best Medication for BPD

In the past, any personality disorder was a death sentence. Now we are learning that BPD in particular has enough commonality to trauma that it can be treated like PTSD.

- Avigail Lev

In this chapter you will learn:

- About the variety of medications available to treat BPD symptoms.

Is There BPD Medication?

Currently, there is no medication created specifically for patients with BPD. However, there are many drugs that can be taken which treat various symptoms of BPD. For example, if you are a person with BPD who frequently experiences anxiety, your doctor may prescribe you anxiety medication to reduce that symptom. What's important to note is that medication is often taken alongside therapy and other treatment, and is not used as the sole treatment for BPD on its own.

85

Patients tend to have mixed views when it comes to taking prescription medication. This could be due to the side effects that many of these medications come with. It is important to discuss your concerns with a doctor and find medication that is suitable for you. Some of the benefits of taking BPD medication are:

- Reduced severity of BPD symptoms.

- Improved daily functioning (such as less work interruptions or conflict in relationships).

- Effectively treating comorbidities that interact with the symptoms of BPD.

- A reduced rate of self-harming behaviors.

As helpful as taking medication can be, it will not necessarily cure BPD. The effectiveness of some medication can also vary from one person to another. For example, depending on the severity of your symptoms, there are some dosages or medications that will not be as effective.

Moreover, if you have multiple medical conditions being treated at the same time, your choice of BPD medication can be limited. For example, if you are currently taking medicine to treat bipolar disorder, it is not advised to take any antidepressants, as they can lead to manic episodes. Speak to your doctor about any co-occurring conditions (even if you suspect that you may have symptoms of another disorder), so that they can offer you the right prescription. It is also recommended to immediately stop taking medication, and seek a doctor, when experience adverse reactions.

Types of Medication to Treat BPD Symptoms

Depending on the BPD symptoms you are experiencing, there are several types of medication available to you. Below are four types of medication common for treating BPD symptoms:

Antidepressants

Antidepressants were originally developed for patients who suffered from mood disorders. However, they are also among the popular types of medication prescribed for BPD. They are particularly effective in BPD patients who simultaneously suffer from anxiety, depression, or emotional reactivity, but they are less effective when treating symptoms of impulsivity or anger.

There are a variety of antidepressants available on the market, although doctors commonly prescribe medication known as selective serotonin reuptake inhibitors (SSRIs). Their job is to adjust the availability of the brain chemical, serotonin. Examples of SSRIs include:

Paxil

Prozac

Zoloft

Celexa

Lexapro

Other less prescribed antidepressants are serotonin-norepinephrine reuptake inhibitors (SNRIs) and monoamine oxidase inhibitors (MAOIs). These types of antidepressants are much older and tend to carry more severe side effects.

Antipsychotics

Some of the first patients to be diagnosed with BPD were prescribed antipsychotic medication. This was because doctors believed that BPD symptoms were bordering between neurosis and psychosis. Nowadays, we understand that BPD does not share many similarities with psychosis, and it technically wouldn't be classified as a psychotic disorder either. However, antipsychotic medication is still effective in treating symptoms like severe mood swings, paranoia, or hostility.

There are two types of antipsychotic medication: typical and atypical antipsychotics. Typical antipsychotics are the more traditional type of medication that are not usually prescribed due to the movement-related side effects they come with. Examples of medication under this category include:

- Navane

- Haldol

- Stelazine

The more commonly prescribed antipsychotics are atypical antipsychotics. These are newer medications that come with less movement-related side effects. Examples include:

- Fanapt

- Caplyta

- Geodon

- Abilify

- Invega

- Rexulti

- Saphris

- Risperdal

- Latuda

- Seroquel

- Zyprexa

- Vraylar

Mood Stabilizers

Mood stabilizers are typically prescribed to treat BPD symptoms like impulsivity and emotion dysregulation. Anticonvulsants, which are medications to treat seizures, are often prescribed to BPD patients due to their mood stabilizing effects. Examples of anticonvulsants include:

- Lamictal

- Trileptal

- Tegretol

- Topamax

- Depakote

- Lithobid

Anti-Anxiety Drugs

For borderline patients who experience intense bouts of anxiety, doctors may prescribe anti-anxiety medication, also called anxiolytics. Unlike other types of medication, there has been little research done to investigate the effectiveness of anti-anxiety drugs in treating BPD-related anxiety. However, on a patient level, there are mixed reviews given about the usefulness of these drugs. Some patients report improvements in their anxiety symptoms, while others report medication like Xanax strengthening their urges to act impulsively.

The most commonly prescribed anti-anxiety medications are benzodiazepines. A few drugs falling under this category include:

- Xanax

- Valium

- Klonopin

- Ativan

The use of benzodiazepines for BPD patients is controversial. Research has shown that in some BPD patients, these medications increase suicidal thinking and impulsivity (Dodds, 2017). There is also a higher risk of patients becoming dependent on benzodiazepines, especially those with known addiction problems, due to their attempts to self-medicate. It is recommended to ask your doctor for non-benzodiazepine anxiolytics.

Chapter Takeaways

In conjunction with psychotherapy, it can be useful to inquire about BPD medication that can reduce some of your more intense symptoms. Speak to your doctor about your options and remember to share your full medical history, including current conditions you are taking medication for. There is no medication that is the best one; each patient will react differently to medication. Find medication that effectively treats *your* symptoms, without causing severe side effects.

The options for treating BPD are endless. Some of the unconventional methods include managing BPD symptoms at home by making healthy lifestyle adjustments. The next chapter will explore some of these alternative BPD remedies.

CHAPTER 9:

At-Home Remedies and Alternative Treatments for BPD

Yet I also recognize this: Even if everyone in the world were to accept me and my illness and validate my pain, unless I can abide myself and be compassionate toward my own distress, I will probably always feel alone and neglected by others.

- Kiera Van Gelder

In this chapter you will learn:

- Natural remedies and techniques that can help you manage BPD symptoms.

Breathwork

The mind-body connection is a powerful phenomenon that explains how your brain or inner world of thoughts and emotions affect your physical health, and vice versa. For example, when you have an anxious thought, you will notice physical discomfort around the chest area caused by an increase in your heart rate. However, the opposite is also true. When your heart is beating uncontrollably, it may trigger your body's natural stress response, which leads to anxious thoughts and feelings.

Think back to what one of the first things you do when you are feeling distressed is. Do you take deep breaths? There is a valid reason for doing this. Taking deep breaths alters your physiology by slowing down your heart rate and allowing more air into your lungs (Russo et al., 2017). But these physiological changes often also lead to reduced feelings of stress and anxiety.

The purpose of breathwork is to induce a state of mental calm by putting your nervous system into a relaxed condition. This process effectively takes your body out of the fight-flight-freeze mode and causes you to feel balanced and emotionally regulated. The more you practice breathwork, the easier it will be to detect when your emotional state is imbalanced. How will you know? You can usually tell by the shortness of your breath, also referred to as "hyperventilating," which allows less oxygen to flow to your lungs.

Breathwork teaches you how to take deeper and longer breaths, so that you can direct your breath to your diaphragm rather than your chest. Longer and deeper breaths put you in a relaxed state of mind because they allow more oxygen into your bloodstream. They also give you a moment to pause and recollect your thoughts to avoid reacting impulsively. Furthermore, research has found that deep breathing is also an effective tool for self-healing (Jahnke, 1999). It improves the flow of lymph fluid throughout the body, which means that immune-boosting cells are able to attack viruses and bacteria a lot quicker.

Below are a few breathing techniques that you can learn and practice whenever you desire to alter your mental and emotional state:

1. Deep Breathing

One of the most basic breathing techniques is deep breathing. The aim of deep breathing is to teach you how to direct your breaths to your stomach and induce a state of relaxation.

To get started, lie down on your bed, facing the ceiling. If you are not at home, you can sit back on a chair and ensure that your spine is lengthened. Place one hand on your stomach and take a deep breath through your nose. You should feel your stomach expanding as the air reaches your diaphragm. When your stomach is filled to capacity, gently purse your lips and release the air slowly out of your mouth. As you do this, you should feel your stomach sinking back to its original position. Continue taking deep breaths for 10 minutes, or until you feel calm.

2. Breath Focus

Breath focus is similar to deep breathing, except, while you are taking deep breaths, your attention is placed on a mental image, word, mantra, etc. This type of exercise can be useful when you are in an anxiety-inducing situation and you need to quickly remind yourself of a positive phrase or statement to keep you calm.

For this technique you won't need to lie down; you can simply close your eyes wherever you are. Take between 3–5 deep breaths, and as you breathe in, bring this image or phrase to your mind. It could be an image of peace or a phrase like, "I am safe". Imagine that you are inhaling this image or phrase in your nose and it fills your entire body. As you exhale, imagine that any undesirable thought or emotion is released out of your mouth. Continue breathing in and out for 10 minutes, or until you feel relaxed.

3. Progressive Muscle Relaxation

This breathing technique induces a state of relaxation by deliberating tensing and releasing specific muscle groups, one at a time. It can also reduce the sensation of pain and ease tension throughout your body.

To get started, lie down on your back and take a few deep breaths. When your body is feeling at ease, take a deep breath and tense your feet muscles. Hold this position for as long as you can hold your breath, then, when you are ready, release the tension and slowly breathe out through your mouth. Continue to do this for all of your muscle groups, working your way up to your neck and face.

You will find that some muscle groups are difficult to physically tense up. In that case, you can imagine holding and releasing tension. For example, when you get to the head, you can imagine concentrating on a strong emotion, like anger, and slowly releasing this emotion as you exhale.

Breath work can significantly improve how you feel throughout the day, especially in difficult moments. Fortunately, you can practice the breathing techniques mentioned above in both private and public spaces, before and during meetings, as well as when you sense a strong urge coming on.

Mindfulness Meditation

Meditation is the practice of quieting the mind to induce a sense of calm and mental clarity. This practice originally comes from Eastern spiritual traditions that date back over 3,000 years; however, Western doctors and researchers have incorporated different types of meditation into mind-body therapeutic interventions.

Mindfulness meditation is one such type of meditation that has been increasingly used by psychologists in their practice. Research has shown that this type of meditation is effective in treating symptoms of various mental illnesses, like anxiety, chronic stress, depression, and BPD (Khoury et al., 2013). What makes mindfulness meditation so effective is the way it encourages awareness. The meditation component helps you slowly quiet the mind and the mindfulness component helps you pay attention to spontaneous thoughts and emotions that arise in the moment.

Dr. Linehan, the psychologist who discovered DBT, is one of the first doctors to incorporate a form of meditation into psychotherapy, especially in the treatment of BPD. She found that this practice helped BPD patients reflect on their thoughts and emotions, instead of reacting impulsively. Mindfulness skills are amongst the many taught in DBT. These skills teach patients how to pause, take a step back, assess the triggering situation without any bias or judgment, and choose the most appropriate response.

Mindfulness meditation is a simple practice that you can learn and carry out at home. Please note that you don't need any previous experience to get started, and each time you sit down and practice meditation, your ability to quiet your mind will become stronger. In general, many beginners set aside between 5–10 minutes for mindfulness meditation. However, you are welcome to select a time frame that works best for you. Below are instructions to practice mindfulness meditation:

- Find a quiet room or area where you can sit alone for the duration of your meditation. Make sure that you are comfortable, either sitting on the floor, lying on a bed, or perched on a chair.

- Body posture is important to release tension and feel relaxed. Whether you are lying down or sitting on a chair, ensure that your neck and spine are lengthened, and your shoulders relaxed.

- Put on a timer for the amount of minutes you will spend in meditation. Doing this will minimize distractions and allow you to fully concentrate on the session.

- Close your eyes and focus on your breathing. You can practice one of the breathing techniques mentioned above, or simply notice the variation of each breath, how deep or shallow your breathing is, etc.

- When you are feeling relaxed, shift your focus to your thoughts. Imagine that you were given VIP access into your own mind, which means that you can observe each thought passing by. Instead of being the "thinker of thoughts" your role has switched to the "witnesser of thoughts".

- As each thought passes by, acknowledge its presence. Look at it and determine what it desires to share with you. Avoid weighing your thoughts as being either good or bad, or suppressing thoughts that you deem inappropriate. See the value in every thought, regardless of its shape and content. Remember to continue breathing deeply, especially as you witness difficult thoughts that might trigger emotions. Use each breath as an anchor to keep you calm and stabilized.

- If you catch yourself becoming preoccupied with a thought, use your breath to gently pull you away from the thought and reestablish yourself as the witness. Continue observing your thoughts until there aren't any more thoughts to witness. If you still have some time left, enjoy this peaceful and 'empty' mental state.

- When the timer goes off, take a few more deep breaths and then open your eyes.

If you are somebody who finds meditation difficult, there are other ways that you can practice mindfulness while still achieving similar outcomes. Below are a few suggestions for turning everyday tasks into mindful moments:

- As you brush your teeth, notice the texture and movement of the brush bristles.

- If you are doing dishes in a sink, take a moment to savor the feeling of warm soapy water on your hands. You can also focus on the sounds of plates and pots as they clank and collide with one another.

- While driving, pay attention to the sound of the engine, the bright colors of the traffic lights, or the vibration coming from your car seat.

- While taking a walk or running on a treadmill, time your breathing with the pace at which you are walking or running. Or, if you are listening to music, use it as a guide for your breathing pattern.

What makes a mindful moment is being fully present in the moment, no matter what you are doing. Train your mind to focus on one task at a time, and devote your time and energy to that task. This kind of intentionality has the same benefit as meditation because of its calming effect.

Getting Enough Sleep

One of the often overlooked symptoms that comes with BPD is sleep disturbances. Generally, sleep problems are not considered to be a defining characteristic of BPD—thus doctors won't always provide treatment with this issue in mind. Nonetheless, studies have investigated the causal relationship between BPD and sleep disturbances and found that BPD patients experience more inconsistency in their sleep times than the general population (Moawad, 2022).

Apart from sleep inconsistencies, people with BPD may also suffer from recurring nightmares. It is estimated that about half of people living with BPD experience recurring nightmares, and, due to this, they are more susceptible to being diagnosed with what is known as nightmare disorder, a condition where patients experience extreme nightmare-related life disruptions (Promises Behavioral Health, 2015). Recurring nightmares can present unique challenges for a person with BPD, such as mental dissociation (detaching from reality) and worsening existing BPD symptoms like anxiety, paranoia, or depression.

One of the symptoms of Hannah's BPD was interrupted sleep. She went to bed at 9p.m., every night, but would twist and turn until the early hours of the morning. What made it harder for her to fall asleep was the bedtime anxiety she would typically experience. Every dark and negative thought would enter her mind, like how much she hated her job or how many more years she had to live. It was usually when everyone was waking up that Hannah could actually fall asleep, but by then she only had about three hours before her morning alarm would ring. With each passing day, her sleep deficit would increase and her energy levels would drop.

Since taking sleeping medication was off the table, Hannah decided that she would make a few lifestyle changes to improve her sleeping routine. The first thing she cut out was coffee. Due to running on low energy, she relied on four cups of coffee per day. However, the caffeine overload was contributing to her lack of sleep. As a substitute for coffee, Hannah increased the fiber in her diet and performed a low-intensity workout four times a week.

The term "sleep hygiene" refers to daily sleeping practices that promote consistent and uninterrupted sleep (Suni, 2022). As someone with BPD, it will take a lot more positive reinforcement to create a sustainable sleeping routine, however, it is possible. Below are some suggestions on how you can improve your sleep hygiene:

1. Create a Sleep Schedule

Train your body to naturally go to sleep and wake up at certain times by enforcing a fixed bedtime and wake-up time. Try to remain consistent even on weekends, so that your body can learn the new sleeping rhythm. Note that you won't always feel tired at your bedtime or fully rested at your waking time. Be patient with the process and give your body enough time to adjust.

2. Avoid Skipping Sleep

It can be tempting to watch another 30 minutes of your favorite show or send a final email minutes before your bedtime. However, doing this shows that sleep isn't one of your priorities. While you might feel full of energy in the evenings, your body needs some time to recharge. The more rested your body is, the less anxiety, fatigue, and irritability you will feel the next day.

3. Create a Bedtime Routine

Preparing for bed hours before you sleep can gently put your mind into a relaxed state. What makes a bedtime routine effective is having a consistent routine of calming activities, performed every night. Your routine might include taking a hot bath, playing soft music, writing in a journal, meditating, switching off electronic devices, drinking chamomile tea, etc. At the beginning, you won't know which activities work best for you, therefore explore various activities before settling on one that is effective in inducing sleep.

4. Be Mindful of Your Lifestyle

Poor sleep hygiene can also be a result of unhealthy lifestyle habits, such as smoking, not getting sufficient natural sunlight, or consuming caffeine or alcohol after 3 p.m. Alcohol consumption might cause you to feel drowsy, but this effect wears off and you are more likely to have light sleep and be woken up at night. Eating dinner too late or consuming heavy meals that take a lot of time and energy for the body to digest can be another cause of insomnia. Healthy lifestyle habits that you can adopt include getting regular physical exercise, reducing highly processed and sugary foods from your diet, and avoiding substances like alcohol or over-the-counter medication that may cause sleep disturbances.

5. Turn Your Bedroom Into a Peaceful Sanctuary

Another factor that we often overlook is how we might feel when going to bed. Ideally, there should be minimal bedroom activities occurring, apart from sex or other relaxing activities. If you live near a busy street, consider devices like ear plugs or white noise machines that can help you drown out as much noise as possible. You can also be intentional about the quality of your bedding and comfort of your mattress and pillows to maximize your rest.

While getting enough sleep is important, so is the quality of your sleep. Good sleep hygiene ensures that your body is fully rested for a fixed number of hours, without any interruptions. What "good sleep hygiene" looks like for each individual will vary, so create sleeping schedules and routines that offer you adequate rest and help you to wake up feeling energized in the mornings.

Chapter Takeaways

You might be a person who prefers to manage your condition using natural remedies that strengthen the mind-body connection. Or, alternatively, these holistic approaches could supplement psychotherapy and other treatment interventions. Either way, the benefit of making mind-body adjustments is that you encourage new habits that can reduce the frequency of stress and hyperarousal, helping you regulate your moods and thoughts naturally.

PART 3:

Building and Maintaining

Relationships With BPD

CHAPTER 10:

Building and Maintaining Healthy Relationships With BPD

A crucial element of the real self is its unconditional acceptance of itself.

\- Michael Adzema

In this chapter you will learn:

- How to educate others about your diagnosis of BPD.

- How to recognize and manage relationship triggers.

How to Describe BPD to Others

After you have received your diagnosis, you will undoubtedly heave a sigh of relief! Finally, you have confirmation that you are not 'crazy', but actually suffer from a real mental condition that affects how you interact with others. It is important to share your diagnosis with close friends and family in order for them to learn how to support you.

Sharing your diagnosis is not easy, especially due to the stigma surrounding BPD. However, by being open about your condition, you are also educating more people about BPD and effectively debunking prevalent myths. Moreover, at a glance, BPD can seem like a case of "acting out" when in reality it is a condition that is more complex in nature.

When describing BPD to others, it can be useful to understand what it is for yourself. Think about how you would describe the condition to someone who has never heard of it before. What are some of the key points you would emphasize? An example of a key point would be explaining the symptoms associated with BPD, and focusing on those that you frequently experience. Out of the nine diagnostic criteria, you might show six symptoms to varying degrees.

After describing what the condition is and the symptoms that you display, you can explain the reality of living with BPD. Think about everyday tasks that you struggle with that the general population is able to complete effortlessly. You can also explain how your symptoms play out in real world scenarios, like how they affect your work or how you respond to stressful situations. What matters most is sharing your truth to the best of your ability. You cannot control how others respond to your explanations (such as whether or not they show sympathy), but you can make it easier for them to understand how you think.

Note that some people may not be able to wrap their minds around the severity of BPD. Perhaps they have never heard about it before or they have no previous experience being in a relationship with someone living with mental illness. The most you can do is describe the physical and emotional impact, making simple analogies and comparisons for them to at least imagine what it might feel like to have BPD. For example, you can compare the intense feeling of rejection to physical chest pains or dissociation to spacing out. This can make your symptoms seem more relatable, thus leading to less speculation.

But sharing the symptoms and daily experience of living with BPD isn't the full story. Truth be told, there are many positive factors that come with this condition. Society as a whole depicts any mental illness as a disadvantage, but if you flip it over and look at it from a different perspective, you can see a handful of advantages. Share some of the positive experiences of having BPD, such as your ability to empathize with others and make them feel accepted or the intensified feelings of love or excitement that make your relationships exhilarating. Being comfortable sharing the positives not only changes perceptions of your condition, but can also help you embrace what sets you apart from others.

Recognizing and Managing Triggers in Relationships

Another important aspect of BPD that you can explain to close friends and family is that your impulsive or extreme behaviors are not deliberate. Unlike most people, you are more likely to feel emotional distress over what seem to be regular words or actions. For example, your romantic partner preparing to leave for work can trigger anxiety. If they aren't aware of your condition, this response can seem uncalled for.

You can also explain to close friends and family how a BPD episode tends to unfold. Since you cannot stop yourself from having these episodes, it can be useful for loved ones to understand what is going through your mind at that vulnerable moment. A typical BPD episode consists of three stages: the trigger, impulsive response, and feelings of guilt and shame.

Stage 1: The Trigger

A trigger is often spontaneous and unpredictable. It can be related to an individual or situation that causes you to feel like attacking, withdrawing, or dissociating from the trigger. A trigger can be related to past experiences, such as being yelled at by a parent, but it can also be activated by deeply rooted fears of rejection or abandonment.

Understanding the impact of past traumas, family upbringing, and attachment style can help you predict certain triggers and act before they become unmanageable. For example, if you are aware that visiting your parents causes you to feel anxious, then you can decide if it might be best to schedule a phone call or video call instead of meeting physically. It might also be useful to create a list of triggers and continue editing your list as you learn new coping skills and habits.

Stage 2: The Impulsive Response

If you are not able to manage your trigger, then it will naturally lead to an impulsive response. This is when you act upon your thoughts or emotions and engage in behaviors that either harm you or others. When you are acting impulsively, it is very difficult to control your actions. It can feel as though you are being guided by pure animal instinct. You may not even remember your actions when you come out of this stage because what you do is largely driven by the fight-flight-freeze response.

It can also be difficult for friends and family to support you during this stage because nothing they say or do will make you calm down, especially if it does not reinforce your preconceived ideas. In intimate relationships, you may push others away, say hurtful words, or accuse them of actions they didn't commit. In general, coming out of this stage will require mindfulness skills, which can help you refocus on the present moment, release you from the strong grip of thoughts and emotions, and regain a sense of control over your mind and body.

Stage 3: Feeling Guilt and Shame

When the storm has passed, your body will slowly calm down. It may take some time before you feel as though you are back to your normal self because a part of you may still feel irritable, numb, or exhausted. The good news is that the trigger doesn't have the same power over you as it did initially. Even something that made you full of rage doesn't move you anymore.

The chronic feeling of emptiness comes sweeping inside your belly. You shift from feeling everything to feeling nothing, not even being aware of activity happening in your environment. It is common to want to spend a few more hours or days alone, not because you desire solitude, but because you don't know how to reconnect with others. A part of you worries if the relationships that were affected during the impulsive behavior are still intact. Another part of you feels regretful for not managing your BPD better. Thoughts about what you have done or what other people think cause significant anxiety.

Due to the symptoms of BPD, your feelings of regret are amplified. In other words, instead of acknowledging what you have done and making amends, you spiral into a storm of self-loathing and shame. If you are not careful, these strong feelings can become a trigger and lead to yet another impulsive response. Psychotherapy can help you work through your feelings of guilt and shame, so that they don't become an obstacle in between you and those you may have hurt. You can learn to not define yourself by your low moments, but rather see yourself as someone who makes mistakes but is courageous enough to own up to them and make the necessary changes.

Coping Strategies to Avoid BPD Rage and Splitting

There will be times when you aren't able to catch your triggers early, and intense anger or splitting may occur. What is important to remember about both anger and splitting is that, once in full effect, it becomes increasingly difficult to control your thoughts and behaviors.

For example, if you have an argument with your romantic partner that triggers a childhood wound, you may start thinking that they are evil or deliberately seek to hurt you. These ideas arise due to sudden splitting and not necessarily what you realistically believe to be true.

While it is tough to feel in control during a BPD episode, there are a few coping strategies that will help you gain more self-awareness and ensure you do the least amount of harm to yourself and others. For example, the moment you recognize an angry thought or anger-related behavior, immediately focus on your breathing. The easiest thing to control before reaching full-blown anger is your breath. You will notice that, due to being triggered, you are more alert and your heart rate might be faster than usual.

Find a quiet room with minimal distractions—or if you can't access a room, sit in your car. Close your eyes and begin taking deep and slow breaths. Continue breathing until the trigger subsides. When you are calm, you can spend a few more minutes journaling about the individual or situation that triggered your anger.

Removing yourself from the source of the trigger is also effective. This isn't an excuse to isolate yourself from others, but instead to retreat to a safe place where you can calm yourself down. You never have to feel obligated to be around other people when you are emotional. Sometimes, the excessive amount of socialization and action in your environment can actually make you feel more anxious and on edge. Take some time to relax by yourself or in the company of people who you feel safe to hang around.

If you are triggered to start the process of splitting, what may be useful is understanding what your brain is thinking. The urge to split occurs when your brain detects a threat. This can be a real or imagined threat, but, to your brain, any threat is treated as being real and dangerous. As a response to this threat, your brain protects you by splitting, giving you enough time to distance yourself from the threatening person or situation.

Being under stress, or experiencing real or perceived rejection and abandonment, can trigger splitting. This means that the relationships that you are the most invested in emotionally are usually those most vulnerable to splitting (meaning that the more vulnerable you are, the greater the risk of rejection and abandonment).

The following coping strategies can give you enough time to adjust your perspective and prevent splitting from taking place:

- Write a list of the positive attributes you most admire in the individual from whom you wish to split.

- Think about five things you are grateful for about the stressful situation you seek to run away from. If any, what lessons have you learned so far?

- Write a list of strengths you most admire about yourself. In your most difficult times, what qualities helped you survive?

- Write down your urges and, next to each one, put an opposite action that you can perform instead. For example, instead of blocking a friend who is bothering you, perhaps you can mute their conversation for a few hours until you feel less reactive.

- If you notice that you are thinking negatively toward someone, interrupt those thoughts with five things you are grateful for about them. Doing this won't excuse what they may have done, it will simply create a more fair assessment of their character.

- To avoid idealizing someone and putting them on a pedestal, practice identifying their strengths and weaknesses. For example, you might admire how supportive your romantic partner is, but also feel frustrated when they don't clean up after themself.

- Write down your urges on paper and tell yourself that you will reassess the urge later on. This will give you time to weigh your decisions before taking action. Remind yourself that you are never in a rush to act on something.

Chapter Takeaways

There is a common myth that people with BPD are not able to maintain good relationships. While it is true that those with BPD need more assistance in the form of psychotherapy to learn interpersonal skills, they are capable of being warm, loving, and supportive friends, family members, and romantic partners. As someone with BPD, it is important to realize that even though you cannot control what triggers you, you can control how you choose to react to it. You can decide to be vigilant about your anger and do your best not to allow it to run rampant in your relationships. The same goes for splitting: You can choose to deliberately see the best in yourself and others, and, even when others disappoint you, to realize that everyone makes mistakes and it doesn't have to define who they are.

Managing relationships with friends and family is often easier than managing relationships with coworkers. Finding the right work environment presents unique challenges to someone with BPD. In the following chapter, we will delve deeper into what those challenges are and how you can overcome them.

CHAPTER 11:

How to Handle Work When You Have BPD

My adopted beliefs were my written script for living, and I played it out like a self-fulfilling prophecy. As I moved toward healing, I learned unconscious patterns can change once brought into awareness.

- Oriana Allen

In this chapter you will learn:

- About the challenges that BPD presents at work.

- What factors to consider when searching for the right job.

- How to handle conflict at work.

Working With BPD

BPD plays a significant role in how you manage the demands of work and your relationships with coworkers. You may have already noticed that living with BPD makes it harder to "fit in" with others, interpret social cues, and remain motivated at work. A common myth about BPD is that those diagnosed with the condition are unable to keep a stable job.

While it is true that BPD symptoms can put a strain on working relationships, they may not show up on a daily basis. In most cases, BPD symptoms tend to flare up when you are stressed or when you get triggered by something, like your boss reprimanding you for poor performance (which could be taken as a sign of rejection). Therefore, it is possible to manage work demands and relationships without experiencing frequent BPD episodes—or quitting your job.

Nevertheless, it may still be difficult to carry out daily work obligations as someone with BPD. The following are challenges unique to employees who are living with BPD:

1. Feeling Different From Others

No matter how inclusive a work culture may be, a person with BPD might feel as though they don't fit in. They desire to settle in and freely express their opinions like other coworkers, but they fear being overly emotional, behaving inappropriately, or facing rejection from others. This feeling of being different can lead to people-pleasing behaviors, like saying 'yes' to every request even when they are overworked. Being excessively generous and available is their way of gaining acceptance from others, but unfortunately this only leads to burnout and boundary violations.

2. All-or-Nothing Thinking

Since people with BPD often live on the extremes, they are more likely to overwork themselves. It isn't uncommon for someone with BPD to answer emails in the evenings, accepting more work than they can manage, and ultimately tiring themselves out until they reach a boiling point. Showing extreme dedication may also be a way to gain validation from coworkers and be seen in a positive light.

3. Splitting

What makes work relationships feel unstable is the all-or-nothing thinking, or splitting, that can be triggered when a person with BPD feels unsafe, criticized, or threatened. For general staff, interactions at work are seen as part of work life, but for someone with BPD, every interaction is taken personally. For example, a bad work review is seen as an attack on their character, rather than constructive feedback. A boss or coworker who voices opinions that are contrary to what the person with BPD believes can be painted as being 'bad' or plotting against them.

4. Doubting Career Choices

Due to having an unstable self-image, someone with BPD may find it difficult to commit to one career path. For the first few months at a job, they might idealize the company and feel excited and settled. However, with great highs come even deeper lows, and within a few months they might be doubting their fit for the job. Their likes and dislikes at work can change from day-to-day, and this may be a constant trigger of frustration or complaining. In extreme cases, their doubt could lead to skipping on promotions, resigning from their position, or behaving in ways that get them fired.

Beth Rees' story paints a realistic picture of how difficult it can be to manage BPD symptoms at work (Rees, 2018):

Things started off well and then, a few months into the role, I had glandular fever and was off work for three months. I couldn't eat, I slept for days and started to get social anxiety through not going outside. When I finally went back, my "phased return" was non-existent and then came the pressure. The days got longer and I was making mistakes at work. I was paranoid and convinced no one liked me. I was pulled aside about the quality of my work and the manager suggested that maybe public relations wasn't for me. I persevered but in the end, I had to choose: either my work improved or I left.

I found another job in a public relations agency back at home and things started off well. Then the same things started happening again; I had brain fog, I felt really spaced out, my work was being done ridiculously slowly and I would cry in the toilets after receiving criticism. I went to see the GP and they said I had depression. I was prescribed medication and when I got back to work, I pulled the manager aside to tell her. She wanted proof in the form of a doctor's note to back up what I was telling her. I got the note from the doctor and carried on with my work.

[...] A week or so later, I met with two managers who asked if I was better yet. I wasn't. We met again a week or two after that, they asked again if I was better and I said I wasn't. They gave me a verbal warning and suggested that I get my act together or I'd be gone. [...] I recently received a diagnosis of borderline personality disorder (emotionally unstable personality disorder) and my new place of work is so supportive and looks out for my well being. It's amazing and I'm very lucky.

What often helps at work is to recognize your BPD symptoms when they flare up. Catching the symptoms early can help you manage your urges and reactions better. It also gives you a moment to assess the source of your trigger and seek assistance from coworkers. Your mental condition can often make you feel like no one at work will understand you, but this isn't true. There are many coworkers who can relate to feeling overwhelmed by work demands or to struggling to accept criticism. Find someone whom you trust at work, who can be your support buddy—and vice versa. Alternatively, you may be better off finding a new job, in a more BPD-friendly environment.

How to Find a BPD-Friendly Job

Highly stressful work environments and BPD are a recipe for disaster! The best kinds of jobs that support BPD are those that offer structure and stability, positive reinforcement, flexible deadlines, and plenty of resources for work support. When looking for the ideal job, consider the following criteria:

1. Work Schedule

A healthy work-life balance is crucial when living with BPD. There will be times when you may need to be hospitalized for BPD-related symptoms or perhaps need time off work to rest. A traditional 9-to-5 job with a fixed number of sick days or leave days may be too restricting. Jobs that offer part-time or flexible work schedules are a better option for you. It is also worth considering the amount of hours of work required each day, and whether you are expected to work day or night shifts (note that evening jobs may disrupt your sleeping schedule).

2. Workplace Environment

The atmosphere or culture at work can also impact your overall moods, motivation, and ability to concentrate on tasks. Depending on the type of BPD you have been diagnosed with, you might prefer working in teams where you can collaborate with others, or you might prefer independent work that doesn't require a lot of interaction with coworkers. If you are somebody who gets bored easily, you may be open to working on multiple tasks or projects, but if challenges make you feel anxious, then you may prefer predictable, routine tasks.

3. Level of Creativity

Some people with BPD work well when they are encouraged to think creatively. Creative work gives them an outlet to express themselves without fear of being judged. However, there are also others living with BPD that feel stressed when required to think out-of-the-box. They prefer to follow instructions, checklists, and standard procedures in order to feel calm and productive. Figure out how much creative freedom you require from a job; this will help you when deciding on the right career fields.

4. Supportive Coworkers

For someone with BPD, daily interactions with people can positively or negatively affect work performance. Unlike other staff, the person with BPD cares about getting along with coworkers, and when there is tension amongst employees (even if they are not part of the conflict), their work morale can be brought low. To avoid the stress of work conflict, finding a company with a strong inclusive and supportive culture is vital. Take some time to read about a company's work policies, how disputes are handled, the code of conduct, and the cultural practices or philosophies that it lives by.

5. Self-Knowledge

Discovering your strengths and weaknesses, skills and passions, can be useful when choosing a career path. For instance, if you know that social interactions are not your strong point, you can look for jobs that can be done independently. There are other factors about yourself that you can consider, such as your values, boundaries, or expectations. Ultimately, the ideal job should help you become the best version of yourself instead of making you feel ashamed of who you are.

Write down a list of strengths, skills, values, passions, and expectations related to work and search for companies that complement who you are.

Strategies to Manage Conflict at Work

When you are living with BPD, you are more sensitive to disagreements at work. When conflict arises, you may have the urge to confront the perceived troublemaker and disarm the situation immediately, or you might dissociate and take a backseat from everything happening. These reactions are typical fight or flight responses that your body relies on to restore a sense of harmony in your environment. However, as the outcomes of these reactions show, you will find that they are ineffective in resolving conflict.

You have an opportunity to rethink how you manage conflict at work and adopt better coping strategies, like communicating assertively, taking ownership of your emotions, and finding win-win solutions. Interpersonal effectiveness and emotion regulation skills, which are taught in DBT, can be helpful in improving the way you respond to disagreements. Below are a few strategies that you can practice when you find yourself in a conflict situation at work:

- **Resist the urge to act on your emotions.** Create a rule that you will only approach those involved in the conflict after you have acknowledged and processed your feelings. Taking action while you are triggered will only cause more harm than good. It is also good to think about the other person's perspective and how they might be feeling as a result of the situation. This will broaden your perspective and ensure that you have a more balanced view about the conflict.

119

- **Look at the bigger picture.** Imagine that the conflict is only a small part of a larger context. What you perceive as being major is actually small and insignificant in the grander scheme of things. Try and see the information that you might be overlooking, the overarching purpose that you have forgotten, or other bigger motivations that have been put to the side.

- **Set intentions for conflict resolution.** Your intentions when resolving conflict are important because they set the tone of the conversation and determine your attitude and behaviors. It should be your intention to walk away from the conversation feeling heard, but also respecting where the other person comes from. You can also set an intention to find a mutual solution, but accept that this may not happen. To manage your fears of rejection and abandonment, try not to personalize everything that you hear; instead listen from a place of understanding, imagining the impact on the other person.

Resolving conflict is never easy. It requires you to face your fears and be vulnerable. Plus, conflict resolution may not always go according to plan. Sometimes, you and the other person may walk away with hurt feelings, rather than being friends. Remember, conflict is a natural part of any relationship. You won't always get along with people or feel understood.

Chapter Takeaways

It is possible to find meaningful work as someone living with BPD, and you shouldn't be scared off by false statements like "people with BPD can't keep a job". However, when choosing the right career path for you, consider factors like the amount of interaction with people, work schedule, the amount of creative freedom, and the support available so you can thrive.

Nevertheless, work life won't be perfect, even when you have found your ideal job. Personality clashes are common in workplaces because teams are made up of unique individuals with different backgrounds and life experiences. Being at odds with others should not be taken as an attack on who you are as a person. Not everybody will be accepting of you, but that is completely fine!

You have learned how to manage relationships with friends, family, and coworkers. However, in the final chapter, we will look at ways that your loved ones can provide greater support to you.

CHAPTER 12:

How to Support Someone With BPD

I understand your pain. Trust me, I do. I've seen people go from the darkest moments in their lives to living a happy, fulfilling life. You can do it too. I believe in you. You are not a burden. You will NEVER BE a burden.

- Sophie Turner

In this chapter you will learn:

- How to support friends and family who are living with BPD.

- What to do when a loved one is self-harming or displaying suicidal behaviors.

Talking to Someone With BPD

When it comes to supporting someone with BPD, how you communicate to them is important. It is not so much *what* you say, but *how* you say it that makes the difference.

As you may know, people with BPD are hypersensitive and they can pick up on subtle nuances in language, defensive body language, and a disapproving tone of voice much easier than other people. The goal of communicating with someone who has BPD is to ensure they feel understood and accepted, even if you are disagreeing with what they are saying or how they are behaving.

A great method to help you communicate effectively is S.E.T., which stands for Support, Empathy, and Truth. This method provides an easy to follow framework for having difficult conversations with your loved one. It allows you to validate their thoughts and feelings while maintaining clear and firm boundaries. This makes it possible to stand up for yourself or express your needs without emotionally injuring the other person. Below is an explanation of each step in the S.E.T. method:

1. Support

When starting a conversation, it is important to express your support for the person with BPD. This can be a short statement like "I love you" or "I want you to know that I am here for you". Starting off with statements like these can disarm the other person and make them more willing to listen to what you have to say. Since people with BPD are sensitive to criticism, showing support from the outset emphasizes that your intentions are good and whatever you say isn't meant to hurt them.

If your loved one responds with a statement suggesting that you don't care about their feelings, it means that they don't feel supported by you. Before you move on to the next step, spend some time conveying your support. You may want to say, "You know I am only a phone call away" or "I will never be too busy to hear you out". If you have shown support in the past, remind them of how and when you have been there for them. This first step should not be overlooked because unless your loved one feels supported, the conversation between you won't feel safe.

2. Empathy

The next step is to express understanding. The purpose here is to validate your loved one's thoughts and feelings. Note that you don't necessarily have to agree with them to accept their views or motivations. Statements like, "I can tell you are frustrated" and "I know this is a lot for you to process right now" are empathetic statements that show you are aware of their emotional experience.

When showing empathy, avoid telling your loved one how they should feel, but instead tell them what you are observing. If they look uncomfortable, let them know that you can see this and it is okay for them to feel that way. If the person with BPD responds by saying you don't understand, it means that they don't register your empathetic feelings. Continue to reinforce your empathetic statements, but in different ways, to show your loved one that you truly get where they are coming from.

3. Truth

After you have shown support and empathy, you can continue by balancing the conversation with truth. Often, the truth is not easy to hear because it can reinforce a boundary, express disagreement, or issue a consequence. Remember, your needs, beliefs, and boundaries are just as important as your loved one's. You never have to compromise on your truth to please or stay in the "good books" of your loved one with BPD.

Being honest about the reality of the situation can also help both of you come to a mutual understanding about what the problem is and how to solve it together. For example, if your loved one is violating your physical space boundary, then you can both objectively look at the situation and create new rules to follow. Truth statements are clear and assertive. They draw a line between what is possible and what is impossible. You might say, "I cannot see you every weekend because I need to make time for myself". You can follow up a truth statement with an alternative solution or suggestion, such as, "I am open to scheduling a 30 minute catch up call on weekends where we cannot meet physically. Would this arrangement work for you?"

Beginning with the support and empathy statements makes the truth less bitter. However, you cannot control how your loved one responds. Remind yourself that they are in charge of managing their response. It is not your responsibility to prevent any negative feelings from erupting. You are only responsible for what you say and how you say it. If your message is clear, empathetic, and honest, then you have done the best you can.

How to Manage a Relationship With a BPD Friend or Family Member

Loving someone with BPD is the same as loving any other imperfect human being. There will be highs and lows, but ultimately what keeps the relationship strong is mutual respect and accepting each other as you are.

Of course, BPD symptoms will sometimes make communication difficult or blow a situation out of proportion—but, you can set healthy boundaries and have go-to coping strategies to protect yourself against being on the receiving end of BPD rage or splitting.

The following coping strategies are just a few that can help you manage your relationship with a friend or family member with

BPD:

1. Learn About BPD

The more you know about BPD, the easier it becomes to tolerate BPD episodes or understand why your loved one thinks or behaves the way they do. Reading this book was a good start, but beyond this, you can learn more about this condition by visiting the following websites:

- **National Education Alliance for Borderline Personality Disorder**: A website that allows loved ones of people with BPD to connect with each other, learn more about BPD through webinars, online courses, audio presentations, and other forms of media. https://www.borderlinepersonalitydisorder.org/

- **Healing From BPD**: A personal blog managed by author Debbie Corsco, who was diagnosed with BPD and now seeks to educate others about the condition. You can find useful articles on the website, including how to practice DBT skills. If you would like to be a supportive BPD community, you are also welcome to join the Facebook group. https://www.my-borderline-personality-disorder.com/

- **Emotions Matter**: A nonprofit organization that aims to increase awareness about BPD, advocate for better treatment options, and help people to cope with the challenges associated with BPD. https://emotionsmatterbpd.org/

It is also important to recognize the impact of BPD symptoms. Having an emotional outburst or making an impulsive decision can be deeply embarrassing for someone with BPD, especially because they are aware that their behavior is socially unacceptable. They do not deliberately try to be difficult or put a strain on their relationships. Understanding that their behaviors are not their fault doesn't mean that you shouldn't hold a loved one accountable; it just means that you are more compassionate and patient with how you approach them.

2. Validate Their Emotions and Experiences

Your loved one with BPD doesn't want special treatment; all they are looking for is acceptance. They want to be reassured that you understand why they feel so strongly about a situation or why they perceived your actions as an attack. You can train yourself to step inside your loved one's shoes and see the world from their perspective. Instead of being quick to take offense about a behavior, you can take a few moments to consider why they thought to behave in that manner. Ask yourself what they could have been thinking at the moment.

Being knowledgeable about BPD symptoms will make it a lot easier to empathize with a loved one. However, remember that not all of their behaviors will be attributed to their condition— they are still human and will have normal reactions to life events too.

3. Schedule Time for Yourself

It is common for a friend or family member with BPD to become the center of attention in the relationship. If you are not careful, you will find yourself investing a lot of your time and energy in making sure they are comfortable in the relationship, while spending little time on yourself.

Healthy relationships are built on reciprocity, which is the natural give-and-take process that occurs between people. Receiving emotional support and being cared for should go both ways. It is

127

okay to ask for help from a loved one with BPD, or to express your thoughts and feelings. When you don't receive the kind of support that you offer your loved one, it is appropriate to sit down with them and have a heart-to-heart. Remind yourself that you are not their caretaker, but an equal in the relationship.

At the same time, don't be shy to set healthy boundaries so you can prioritize your own needs. Practicing self-care is what gives you enough energy to show up for your friends and family. Some of the best self-care practices don't even require spending money. It could be as simple as taking 15 minutes in the morning to journal, meditate, pray, or recite affirmations. You might also set personal goals for yourself and dedicate time in your schedule to work on those goals. Your life is bigger than any relationship and you deserve to invest your time in other meaningful pursuits.

4. Stop Making Excuses for Your Loved One

It is difficult not to sympathize with your loved one's mental disorder and the various ways it impacts their life. However, it is important to remind yourself that they are capable of having a meaningful life like anybody else. Being diagnosed with BPD doesn't make them vulnerable to the extent that they cannot tell right from wrong or maintain relationships without your help. People with BPD are intelligent, talented, and highly-functioning individuals who don't need to be rescued.

When your loved one has a BPD episode, take a step back and allow them to feel whatever they want to feel. Your job is to simply validate their experience, not solve their problems for them. If your loved one's behaviors lead to unpleasant consequences, allow them to experience the consequences so they can learn from the situation. Sometimes, the best way you can show your support is to stand on the sidelines and cheer for them as they go through the ups and downs of life. This shows that you trust them to make good choices for their life and bounce back from setbacks.

5. Reinforce Healthy Boundaries

In order to make a relationship feel safe with a BPD friend or family member, you need to create structure with set norms and expectations. Your loved one might challenge the norms and expectations, but deep down their nervous system will thank you for it! Healthy boundaries are a great tool to set limits in the relationship and clearly define acceptable and unacceptable behavior. Boundaries are not supposed to be a form of punishment, but rather a guideline on how to treat each other.

Both of you come into the relationship with needs and desires, and healthy boundaries ensure that your needs are honored. A lack of boundaries might open your relationship to manipulative or abusive behaviors that will eventually damage the level of trust and safety between you. Setting and enforcing healthy boundaries can also help your loved one learn how to regulate their emotions and behaviors better. In a way, the boundaries become standards that they seek to maintain in order to create harmony in the relationship. Examples of boundaries that you can set include:

- Walking away from a conversation when the other person raises their voice or insults you.

- Responding to personal text messages only before or after working hours.

- Requesting 24 hours to process a request and provide an answer.

- Ending phone calls after 30 minutes.

- Having two weekends a month to yourself.

Note that there are some boundaries that can be held loosely and compromise can be reached. However, there are also boundaries that are non-negotiables, meaning that you hold strongly to the standard that you have set and cannot compromise. Be clear about your loose and non-negotiable boundaries so you can avoid push back.

6. Encourage Your Loved One to Seek Treatment

It can be tempting to become your loved one's voice of reason or unofficial therapist because you understand them better than anyone else. However, playing the role of therapist can harm your relationship since it prevents you from truly connecting on matters unrelated to your loved one's condition. Educate yourself on some of the effective BPD treatments available and recommend these to your loved one. Remind them that you are not qualified to teach them some of the vital coping skills required to manage their condition.

As much as you care about them, there are licensed therapists who are better suited to mentor and guide them on their healing path. There are also some forms of therapy, like family or couple's therapy, which you can attend with your loved one. These therapies can help you strengthen your communication skills and become more responsive to each other's needs.

Supporting a Loved One Who Is Suicidal

The thought that your loved one may be suicidal can be terrifying. If you could, you would somehow take on the emotional pain they are carrying—but you can't, and this leaves you feeling hopeless. But, the truth is that there is something you can do and it begins with educating yourself about suicidal thoughts and behaviors.

Suicide rates have increased over the years due to a number of factors, like the growing rate of people diagnosed with mental illnesses. According to Suicide Awareness Voices of Education (SAVE), suicide ranks 12th in the leading causes of death in the U.S. Everyday, an average of 125 Americans die at the hands of suicide, and for every suicide death, there are about 25 suicide attempts (SAVE, 2020). This means that suspicions that your loved one may be suicidal should be taken seriously and reacted to immediately.

One of the myths that must be debunked is that a suicidal person who suffers from BPD is seeking attention. When someone suggests that they don't want to live anymore or that they wish they could die, they are actually crying out for help. This is the best time to lean in to your loved one and show them through actions that they are valued and cared for. Psychologist Ursula Whiteside believes that strengthening the connection you have with a suicidal loved one reduces the risk of suicide (Chatterjee, 2020). This is because they recognize that they belong, and this sense of belonging can bring about greater resilience. Plus, the earlier you intervene and show care, the less your loved one feels alone.

There are numerous ways you can support a suicidal person. Below are four that can make a significant difference:

Recognize the Warning Signs

It is important to understand where a loved one's suicidal thoughts and behaviors come from. In other words, try to be involved in their lives enough to identify harmful patterns of behavior that may be triggered by mental illness, substance abuse, trauma, or other stressful life events. Below are a few risk factors that make a person vulnerable to suicide:

- History of attempted suicide
- Mental disorders like BPD, schizophrenia, bipolar disorder, anxiety disorders, or depression
- Chronic or terminal illness
- Financial problems
- Substance abuse problems
- Limited access to healthcare services
- Access to self-harming tools and medication
- Expressed feelings of hopelessness

If your loved one has been exposed to any of these risk factors, then it is crucial to remain on high alert. Monitor their speech, routines, and lifestyle choices to assess their mental health. Some of the behavioral warning signs to look out for include:

- Recurring mood swings
- Sudden calmness after a depressive episode
- Isolating from others
- Loss of interest in social activities they used to enjoy
- Poor sleeping patterns, hygiene, and grooming
- Being in a state of deep despair (seeing no reason to continue living)
- Making preparations like searching for self-harming tools or getting their affairs in order
- Threatening to commit suicide

Reach Out With Compassion

When you notice a change in someone, reach out to them and see how they are doing. For some people, seeking support makes them feel desperate, so they would appreciate close friends and family stepping up and approaching them. As you have read here, one of the symptoms of BPD is the fear of abandonment. Your loved one who is contemplating suicide may be suffering from real or perceived loneliness. Reaching out to them shows that there is at least one person who they matter to, and this can reduce their sense of being abandoned.

When reaching out, you can simply make casual conversation. It isn't necessary to bring up your concerns, although if you have established a sense of safety in your relationship, you certainly can. You can use the S.E.T. method mentioned above when sharing your concerns with a loved one.

Assess the Level of Risk

The default response when someone you care about threatens suicide is to panic, however this won't help you manage the situation. Your mind and body should be calm because you need to think clearly and logically. Before you take any action, the first step will be to assess the level of risk. Not everybody who expresses suicidal thoughts needs to be sent to the emergency room.

In fact, research has shown that many who have suicidal thoughts don't experience the kind of impulsive thought that leads to an actual suicide attempt (Chatterjee, 2020). Asking your loved one how strong their urges are, or for how long they have been having these thoughts, can help you gauge the level of risk. If you are looking for a more structured tool to assess your loved one's risk level, you can use the suicide severity scale, known as the Columbia Protocol, created by psychiatrists at Columbia University (The Columbia Lighthouse Project, n.d.).

When you determine that your loved one is at a high risk of suicide, you will need to buy time. In many cases, strong urges to commit suicide often subside (or become manageable) within 24–48 hours. Buying time will also give you a chance to make the necessary preparations to seek medical assistance. If possible, stay with your loved one so that you can monitor the minute-by-minute changes in their mood and provide constant validation and a calming atmosphere. Ask them if they have any self-harming tools on hand and remove these from their environment. It may also be useful to ask them to take a few days or weeks off electronic devices and social media.

Help Your Loved One Create a Safety Plan

When you have successfully managed the risk level and your loved one is feeling less triggered to follow through with their suicide attempt, sit down with them and discuss ways of preventing this crisis in the future. If you are unable to have this kind of conversation with them, you can seek the help of a licensed therapist.

Research has shown that having a safety plan reduces the risk of suicide and provides healthy coping strategies to turn to when that urge to self-harm arises. The American Foundation for Suicide Prevention provides an online template to create a solid safety plan. Some of the components of the plan include writing down common triggers, helpful coping strategies and distractions, as well as people to reach out to for support (Vibrant Emotional Health, n.d.).

If your loved one doesn't have access to healthcare, you can search for digital tools and online support that they can turn to. For example, they can download apps like Calm or Virtual Hope Box that teach useful coping techniques. There are also many support forums and blogs run by suicide survivors that provide a safe place to talk about everyday life struggles. Showing your loved one that plenty of help is available—and many of it is free—can be empowering for them!

Chapter Takeaways

Supporting a loved one with BPD requires a gentle approach. You need to momentarily forget about your own preconceived ideas and step inside their shoes. Look at the world from their perspective and recognize why they think and behave the way they do. Validation is key when communicating and showing support to someone with BPD. This doesn't mean agreeing with them or letting them get away with disruptive behavior, but rather showing them that you understand where they are coming from. It is also important to reinforce the message that you are not going to leave them, but you will hold them accountable for their actions.

However, there is a point where your support becomes insufficient and your loved one needs medical assistance. For instance, only a licensed therapist is able to teach someone with BPD coping skills to manage their condition. Don't be afraid to reach out for medical support when it becomes necessary.

If you suspect that a loved one may be battling with suicidal thoughts and behaviors, here are a few ways to seek help:

- Call the suicide prevention hotline/crisis hotline at 1-800-273-8255.

- Text 'START' to 741741.
- Call 911 if in immediate danger.

Conclusion

Though it may not seem like it at times, I'm really doing the best I can.

- Mick Goodman

BPD is historically and presently one of the most misunderstood mental disorders in the world. This is seen in the widespread misinformation about and misdiagnoses of the condition. However, we can celebrate the fact that doctors are beginning to give this condition the attention that it deserves and investigating treatments that provide relief.

When it was first discovered, BPD was seen as being an illness bordering neurosis and psychosis. Nowadays, we know that it is not a type of psychosis, but rather a personality disorder that affects how people see themselves and relate to others. None of the symptoms displayed by BPD patients are intentional, even though to someone who doesn't know much about the condition it may seem that way. We still have a long way to go in educating society about people with BPD and the kinds of health, identity, work, and relationship challenges they experience on a daily basis.

The purpose of this book was to provide you with a comprehensive introduction into BPD and what makes it so unique from other personality disorders. Unfortunately, when my mother was misdiagnosed with bipolar disorder, books like these weren't available. It is my wish that you or your loved ones who might be showing signs of BPD find answers to some of your burning questions by flipping through these pages. BPD is no longer a mystery or an untreatable condition, as some medical professionals used to think. There are a multitude of ways to manage symptoms, build and maintain healthy relationships, and thrive as someone living with BPD.

As a parting message, remember that you are not alone. You might be the only one in your family, friendship circle, or workplace with BPD, but I guarantee you that there are millions of people across the world who can relate to your experiences. The stories provided throughout this book are proof that there are many fighting the same symptoms that you fight on a daily basis. Find online communities with like-minded people. Talk about your experiences and gain strength from those who have overcome what you are currently going through.

While physical, medical, and community support is available, you must be willing to seek it. Take charge of your health and do the best that you can to prevent your BPD from placing restrictions on your life.

And, if you have found this book useful, please leave a review.

Thank You

I really appreciate you buying and finishing this book. I'm SO THANKFUL for your support and hope this book has been beneficial to you.

There are numerous books on this subject, so I'm grateful and appreciative that you chose this one.

Before you go, I wanted to ask you for one last small favor. **It would be very helpful to me if you considered leaving a review on the platform. One of the best and simplest ways to support books from independent authors like me is to leave a review.**

Your opinions are very valuable to me. I'll be able to support other readers by continuing to write books like this. To hear from you would mean so much. I read every single review submitted.

References

A breakthrough for borderline personalities: Dialectical Behavior Therapy proves effective. (2011, May 10). Promises Behavioral Health. https://www.promises.com/addiction-blog/dialectical-behavior-therapy-proves-effective-for-borderline-personalities/

A guide to transference-focused psychotherapy. (2022, February 11). McLean Hospital. https://www.mcleanhospital.org/essential/tfp

About the Protocol The Columbia Lighthouse Project. (n.d.). The Columbia Lighthouse Project. https://cssrs.columbia.edu/the-columbia-scale-c-ssrs/about-the-scale/

American Sleep Association. (2019, September 9). Sleep hygiene tips - Research and treatments. American Sleep Association. https://www.sleepassociation.org/about-sleep/sleep-hygiene-tips/

Antonatos, L. (2022, June 29). Borderline rage: What it is, triggers and how to manage. Choosing Therapy. https://www.choosingtherapy.com/borderline-rage/

Best jobs for people with borderline personality disorder (BPD)? (2022, March 24). PsychReel. https://psychreel.com/best-jobs-for-people-with-borderline-personality-disorder-bpd/

Borderline Personality Disorder quotes (74 quotes). (n.d.-a). Goodreads. Retrieved August 3, 2022, from https://www.goodreads.com/quotes/tag/borderline-personality-disorder#:~:text=%E2%80%9CI

Boudin, M. (2022, June 29). 17 Quotes about BPD. Choosing Therapy. https://www.choosingtherapy.com/bpd-quotes/

BPD impacts my life in every way. (2021, May 25). Rethink. https://www.rethink.org/news-and-stories/blogs/2021/05/bpd-impacts-my-life-in-every-way-gabby-s-story/

Buffum Taylor, R. (2022, April 1). Dialectical Behavioral Therapy. WebMD. https://www.webmd.com/mental-health/dialectical-behavioral-therapy

Canadian Mental Health Association. (2015). What's the difference between CBT and DBT? Here To Help. https://www.heretohelp.bc.ca/q-and-a/whats-the-difference-between-cbt-and-dbt

Chatterjee, R. (2020, December 15). Reach out: How to help someone at risk of suicide. NPR. https://www.npr.org/sections/health-shots/2019/04/20/707686101/how-to-help-someone-at-risk-of-suicide

Cherney, K. (2022, July 13). Quiet BPD: Symptoms, causes, diagnosis and treatment. Healthline. https://www.healthline.com/health/quiet-bpd

Cherry, K. (2022, February 22). Mindfulness meditation. Verywell Mind. https://www.verywellmind.com/mindfulness-meditation-88369

Clarkin, J. F., Foelsch, P. A., Levy, K. N., Hull, J. W., Delaney, J. C., & Kernberg, O. F. (2001). The development of a psychodynamic treatment for patients with borderline personality disorder: A preliminary study of behavioral change. Journal of Personality Disorders, 15(6), 487–495. https://doi.org/10.1521/pedi.15.6.487.19190

141

Clarkin, J. F., Levy, K. N., Lenzenweger, M. F., & Kernberg, O. F. (2007). Evaluating three treatments for borderline personality disorder: A multiwave study. American Journal of Psychiatry, 164(6), 922–928. https://doi.org/10.1176/ajp.2007.164.6.922

Diagnosis - Borderline personality disorder. (2021, February 12). NHS. https://www.nhs.uk/mental-health/conditions/borderline-personality-disorder/diagnosis/

DBT skills list. (n.d.-a). DBT Self Help. https://dbtselfhelp.com/dbt-skills-list/

Dialectical Behavior Therapy (DBT): What it is and purpose. (2022c, April 19). Cleveland Clinic. https://my.clevelandclinic.org/health/treatments/22838-dialectical-behavior-therapy-dbt

Distract with Wise Mind ACCEPTS. (n.d.-b). DBT Self Help. https://dbtselfhelp.com/dbt-skills-list/distress-tolerance/accepts/

Dodds, T. J. (2017). Prescribed benzodiazepines and suicide risk. The Primary Care Companion for CNS Disorders, 19(2). https://doi.org/10.4088/pcc.16r02037

Fowler, P. (2022, January 17). Breathing techniques for stress relief. WebMD. https://www.webmd.com/balance/stress-management/stress-relief-breathing-techniques

Grinker, R. R., Werble, B., & Drye, R. C. (1968). The borderline syndrome : A behavioral study of ego functions. Basic Books.

Guarnotta, E. (2022, June 22). What is a petulant borderline? 10 Signs and how to get help. Choosing Therapy. https://www.choosingtherapy.com/petulant-borderline/

Gunderson, J. G., & Hoffman, P. D. (2016). Beyond borderline

: True stories of recovery from borderline personality disorder. New Harbinger Publications, Inc.

Hancock, C. (2017, June 28). The stigma associated with Borderline Personality Disorder. NAMI. https://www.nami.org/Blogs/NAMI-Blog/June-2017/The-Stigma-Associated-with-Borderline-Personality

Hempel, R. J. (2019, December 2). Using radically open dialectical behavior therapy (RO DBT) to treat problems of overcontrol. Psychology Tools. https://www.psychologytools.com/articles/using-radically-open-dialectical-behavior-therapy-ro-dbt-to-treat-problems-of-overcontrol/

Holly, K. J. (2020, April 16). Borderline personality disorder quotes. Healthy Place. https://www.healthyplace.com/insight/quotes/borderline-personality-disorder-quotes#:~:text=%22Having%20borderline%20feels%20like%20eternal

Houghton, B. (2018, April 18). The 3 stages of my borderline personality disorder episodes. The Mighty. https://themighty.com/topic/borderline-personality-disorder/stages-of-bpd-episodes-borderline-personality-disorder

Jahnke, R. (1999). The healer within : Using traditional Chinese techniques to release your body's medicine. Harperone.

Jameson, L. (2018, July 1). What it's like to have rage "blackouts" when you live with borderline personality disorder. Yahoo. https://www.yahoo.com/lifestyle/apos-rage-apos-blackouts-apos-203620235.html

Jarvis, J. (2016, July 15). When someone with borderline

personality disorder "cries wolf". The Mighty.
https://themighty.com/topic/borderline-personality-
disorder/borderline-personality-disorder-and-attention-seeking

Johnston, E. (2019). How the SET method improves
communication for people with BPD. Verywell Mind.
https://www.verywellmind.com/support-empathy-truth-set-for-
borderline-personality-425229

Johnston, E. (2021, March 20). Take a break from confrontation
and give yourself time to reflect. Verywell Mind.
https://www.verywellmind.com/taking-a-break-from-
confrontation-425164

Khoury, B., Lecomte, T., Fortin, G., Masse, M., Therien, P.,
Bouchard, V., Chapleau, M.-A., Paquin, K., & Hofmann, S. G.
(2013). Mindfulness-based therapy: A comprehensive meta-
analysis. Clinical Psychology Review, 33(6), 763–771.
https://doi.org/10.1016/j.cpr.2013.05.005

Kvarnstrom, E. (2018, January 5). How do you love someone
with borderline personality disorder? Bridges to Recovery.
https://www.bridgestorecovery.com/blog/love-someone-
borderline-personality-disorder/

Lavender, N. J. (2013, October 16). Do you know the 4 types of
borderline personality disorder? Psychology Today.
https://www.psychologytoday.com/za/blog/impossible-
please/201310/do-you-know-the-4-types-borderline-
personality-disorder

LifeStance Health. (2019, October 7). How to love someone
with a borderline personality disorder. Georgia Behavioral
Health Professionals. https://www.mygbhp.com/blog/loving-
someone-borderline-personality-disorder/

Living inside the mind of borderline personality disorder. (2017, June 8). Avalon Malibu. https://www.avalonmalibu.com/blog/this-is-what-its-like-to-live-inside-the-mind-of-borderline-personality-disorder/

Lo, I. (2021, July 23). The struggles of quiet BPD. Psychology Today. https://www.psychologytoday.com/za/blog/living-emotional-intensity/202107/the-struggles-quiet-bpd

Madeson, M. (2022, June 10). Mentalization-based therapy guide: Best worksheets and techniques. Positive Psychology. https://positivepsychology.com/mentalization-based-therapy/

Mae, K. (2019, March 4). How I cope with "splitting" because of borderline personality disorder. The Mighty. https://themighty.com/topic/borderline-personality-disorder/how-to-cope-with-splitting-borderline-personality-disorder

Marsha M. Linehan quote. (n.d.-b). Goodreads. https://www.goodreads.com/author/show/202733.Marsha_M_L inehan

Mattocks, N. (2019, October 11). Borderline personality disorder myths and facts. NAMI. https://nami.org/Blogs/NAMI-Blog/October-2019/Borderline-Personality-Disorder-Myths-and-Facts

McHaffie, H. (2020, April 23). Living and working with BPD - A navigational guide. Independent Cinema Office. https://www.independentcinemaoffice.org.uk/blog-living-and-working-with-bpd-a-navigational-guide/

Miller, K. (2019, June 19). CBT explained: An overview and summary of CBT (Incl. History). Positive Psychology. https://positivepsychology.com/cbt/

Millon, T., & Davis, R. (1996). Disorders of personality : DSM-IV and beyond. Wiley.

Moawad, H. (2022, January 27). Sleep patterns in borderline personality disorder. Psychiatric Times. https://www.psychiatrictimes.com/view/sleep-patterns-in-borderline-personality-disorder

Motivational and inspirational quotes. (2021, August 18). Borderline Support UK. https://borderlinesupport.org.uk/recovery/quotes/

Myths about borderline personality disorder. (2022, May 26). The Recovery Village. https://www.therecoveryvillage.com/mental-health/borderline-personality-disorder/bpd-myths/

Nestler, A. (2020, February 17). The underdiagnosed (and misunderstood) type of borderline personality disorder. The Mighty. https://themighty.com/topic/borderline-personality-disorder/underdiagnosed-type-borderline-personality-disorder-discouraged

Nestler, A. (2021, October 29). How to describe borderline personality disorder to those who don't understand. NAMI. https://www.nami.org/Blogs/NAMI-Blog/October-2021/How-to-Describe-Borderline-Personality-Disorder-to-Those-Who-Don-t-Understand#:~:text=Give%20Specific%20Information%20About%20the%20Disorder&text=A%20pattern%20of%20unstable%20and

Nightmares have unique, damaging impact on BPD sufferers. (2015, April 21). Promises Behavioral Health. https://www.promises.com/addiction-blog/nightmares-have-unique-damaging-impact-on-bpd-sufferers/

Norah Vincent quote. (n.d.-c). Goodreads. https://www.goodreads.com/author/show/16532.Norah_Vincent

Pelham, V. (2021, May 27). What to do when a loved one is suicidal. Cedars-Sinai. https://www.cedars-sinai.org/blog/when-a-loved-one-is-suicidal.html

Personality disorders. Annabelle Psychology (Clinical Psychologists). https://www.annabellepsychology.com/psychotherapy

Personality disorder. (2022a, April 16). Cleveland Clinic. https://my.clevelandclinic.org/health/diseases/9636-personality-disorders-overview

Personality disorders - Symptoms and causes. (n.d.). Mayo Clinic. https://www.mayoclinic.org/diseases-conditions/personality-disorders/symptoms-causes/syc-20354463#:~:text=A%20personality%20disorder%20is%20a

Personality disorders: Types, causes, symptoms and treatment. (2022b, April 16). Cleveland Clinic. https://my.clevelandclinic.org/health/diseases/9636-personality-disorders-overview#:~:text=Approximately%209%25%20of%20adults%20in

Raypole, C. (2019a, January 25). Dialectical Behavioral Therapy (DBT). Healthline Media. https://www.healthline.com/health/dbt#skills

Raypole, C. (2019b, March 8). Schema therapy: Theory, schemas, modes, goals, and more. Healthline. https://www.healthline.com/health/schema-therapy-2#find-a-therapist

Rees, B. (2018, March 22). Borderline personality disorder in the workplace. Mind. https://www.mind.org.uk/information-support/your-stories/borderline-personality-disorder-in-the-workplace/

Renée Knight quote. (n.d.-d). Goodreads. https://www.goodreads.com/author/show/8074596.Ren_e_Knig ht

Ruggero, C. J., Zimmerman, M., Chelminski, I., & Young, D. (2010). Borderline personality disorder and the misdiagnosis of bipolar disorder. Journal of Psychiatric Research, 44(6), 405–408. https://doi.org/10.1016/j.jpsychires.2009.09.011

Russo, M. A., Santarelli, D. M., & O'Rourke, D. (2017). The physiological effects of slow breathing in the healthy human. Breathe, 13(4), 298–309. https://doi.org/10.1183/20734735.009817

Salters-Pedneault, K. (2020a, April 22). How mindfulness meditation can help borderline personality disorder. Verywell Mind. https://www.verywellmind.com/mindfulness-meditation-for-living-with-bpd-425382

Salters-Pedneault, K. (2020b, November 9). How grounding exercises can help you cope with BPD symptoms. Verywell Mind. https://www.verywellmind.com/grounding-exercises-425376

Salters-Pedneault, K. (2020c, December 1). How the stigma of BPD can lead to a misdiagnosis and wrong treatment. Verywell Mind. https://www.verywellmind.com/stigma-a-definition-of-stigma-425329

Salters-Pedneault, K. (2021a, November 9). 9 Symptoms may indicate borderline personality disorder diagnosis. Verywell Mind. https://www.verywellmind.com/borderline-personality-disorder-diagnosis-425174

Salters-Pedneault, K. (2021b, November 30). What to expect during a borderline personality disorder assessment. Verywell Mind. https://www.verywellmind.com/bpd-assessment-process-what-to-expect-425173

Salters-Pedneault, K. (2022, February 14). Borderline personality disorder medications can treat symptoms. Verywell Mind. https://www.verywellmind.com/borderline-personality-disorder-medications-425450

Saxena, S. (2022, June 21). Cognitive behavioral therapy for borderline personality disorder. Choosing Therapy. https://www.choosingtherapy.com/cbt-for-bpd/

Scott, J. (2017, July 8). How borderline personality disorder complicates my insomnia. The Mighty. https://themighty.com/topic/insomnia/borderline-personality-disorder-bpd-insomnia

Smith, M., & Segal, J. (2021, October). Borderline personality disorder (BPD). Help Guide. https://www.helpguide.org/articles/mental-disorders/borderline-personality-disorder.htm

Suicide statistics and facts. (2020). SAVE. https://save.org/about-suicide/suicide-statistics/

Suicidal behavior & signs. (2017). Cleveland Clinic. https://my.clevelandclinic.org/health/articles/11352-recognizing-suicidal-behavior

Suni, E. (2022, August 9). What is sleep hygiene? Sleep Foundation. https://www.sleepfoundation.org/sleep-hygiene

The history of BPD. (2014b, August 25). Optimum Performance Institute.

https://www.optimumperformanceinstitute.com/bpd-treatment/the-history-of-bpd/

Tricaso, K. (2021, March 2). 8 Ways to identify quiet borderline personality disorder. Modern Intimacy. https://www.modernintimacy.com/8-ways-to-identify-quiet-borderline-personality-disorder/

V, J. (2018, March 28). 29 Ways people with borderline personality disorder self-sabotage. The Mighty. https://themighty.com/topic/borderline-personality-disorder/bpd-borderline-personality-disorder-self-sabotage

Vibrant Emotional Health. (n.d.). My Safety Plan. https://www.mysafetyplan.org/

Vogel, K. (2022, March 3). How can breathing rhythms affect your emotions? Psych Central. https://psychcentral.com/lib/change-how-you-feel-change-how-you-breathe#emotions-affect-the-breath

What causes personality disorders? (2022, January). Mind. https://www.mind.org.uk/information-support/types-of-mental-health-problems/personality-disorders/causes/

What goes on in the mind of someone with borderline? (2018, May 14). The Guest House. https://www.theguesthouseocala.com/what-goes-on-in-the-mind-of-someone-with-borderline/

What is discouraged borderline personality disorder? (2014a, August 18). Optimum Performance Institute. https://www.optimumperformanceinstitute.com/bpd-treatment/discouraged-borderline-personality-disorder/

What is impulsive borderline personality disorder? (2017, August 18). Optimum Performance Institute.

https://www.optimumperformanceinstitute.com/bpd-treatment/impulsive-borderline-personality-disorder/

Made in United States
North Haven, CT
07 August 2023

40081372R00096